From Illness to Wellness

The Innovative Healthcare Approach

Dr. Robert Abraham, D.C., C.C.I.P

First Edition

Printed in the U.S.A.
ISBN-13: 978-1717139849
ISBN-10: 1717139841

Table of Contents

Dedication

To my family,

I will never be able to put into words my appreciation for what you have done for me. You have always stood by and supported me through the good and bad times. You never lost faith in me. There is no way I can pay you back for all you have done and I would not be where I am today if it was not for you. Dad, I treat every patient with you in mind; wishing I could have known what I know today when you were going through your health issues.

To my wife, Sara:

You've always accepted me for who I am and support my hustle as I chase my dreams. I will never forget your sacrifices and support. I love you.

To my partners, Joel, Mark and Ron:

Thank you for believing in me and my vision. Thank you for your constant support. I look forward to continued success and changing more and more lives everyday.

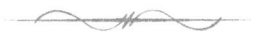

About Dr. Robert Abraham

Deciding on the Natural Healing Path

I am an Oviedo local and have lived in our lovely town since 1999. My father's back troubles were what led me to explore the chiropractic profession. The first back surgery my dad received took place when I was nine. There were two more surgeries by the time I entered chiropractic school. I watched my father go through multiple procedures, see numerous doctors and surgeons, take medications and try to endure the difficult healing process post-surgery, only to experience temporary relief and suffer from the short-term and long-term complications of surgery.

I believe that if my father had known about chiropractic care before he elected to have surgery, his life would be significantly different. It has become my passion to educate people about what chiropractic can do for them and how it can potentially change their lives.

I worked as a pharmaceutical courier while studying at UCF. My job was to deliver medications from pharmacies to nursing homes and assisted living facilities. I saw how poor the quality of life was for most of the individuals living there and neuropathy and weight gain were the main reasons. I also saw the terrible addictions to prescription drugs and the dependency and numbness they caused. This was a major turning point in my life because from this experience stemmed my interest in chiropractic care and my turning away from the traditional medical model and the "sick-care" system it takes full advantage of.

Providing Effective Health Care

A statistic states that only 10% of the population has seen a chiropractor. I couldn't help but imagine what would have been different if the message of chiropractic had reached my father before he opted for surgery. I wanted to impact people before they got to that vulnerable point and was motivated to join the chiropractic profession.

To begin my chiropractic education, I attended the University of Central Florida and graduated with a Bachelor of Science in Health Sciences. I then enrolled at Palmer College of Chiropractic in Port Orange, FL and earned my Doctor of Chiropractic degree. I graduated both institutions with honors. I have successfully completed all four parts of the National Chiropractic Board of Examiners. I am also a proud member of the American Chiropractic Association and The Florida Chiropractic Association.

Enjoying Life in Oviedo

In my spare time, I like to spend time with my family. My lovely wife is from Clearwater, FL and has moved here with me to open CryoNext Integrative Healthcare in our growing area. It is important to me to give back to the community I grew up in. I have coached basketball and soccer since my undergraduate days, being a mentor for local area children. I am involved in my church and enjoy attending local health and wellness events, as well as staying active and playing basketball and soccer in our local leagues.

CryoNext Integrative Healthcare

CryoNext Integrative Healthcare is a multi-disciplinary medical facility that combines chiropractic, medical, rehabilitative and regenerative services, along with the best and latest in modalities. It was founded in by Dr. Robert Abraham in 2016 with the first location in Oviedo. A second location is now open in Lake Nona. Our health care centers are both conveniently located off the 417, easy to reach from all the surrounding communities.

Our team's mission is to offer the most uniquely individualized and professional care available and to promote the wellbeing of all patients, while helping each achieve and maintain the highest quality of life. We also strive to provide cutting-edge, state-of-the-art modalities and services to our Central Florida communities.

Performance Medicine Solutions

Our practice name stems from the integrative healthcare and medicine model and the collaboration of all the best and latest in healthcare technology. One of those technologies is whole body cryotherapy and the numerous benefits it offers. In our facilities, you can find chiropractic care, whole body cryotherapy, stem cell therapy, platelet-rich plasma therapy, LED light therapy, compression therapy, cupping and Kinesio Taping®. Many of these services cannot be found elsewhere in the area or even the state.

CryoNext Integrative Healthcare is an integrative health care center where you can benefit from our broad array of services. We seek to assist you in improving your performance in life, boosting your well-being with nonsurgical, drug-free solutions. Medicine is ever-changing and with the constant development of new technologies, the possibilities are endless. At CryoNext Integrative Healthcare, we have collaborated with industry leaders and experts to bring the most cutting-edge treatment options to our facilities right here in Central Florida.

Train The Mind. The Body Will Follow.

There are many different aspects to being healthy and none can be compromised. With so many options available, we can help you discover true health. Our team includes a chiropractor, nurse practitioner and medical doctor in addition to our highly qualified, knowledgeable support staff.

Ultimately, we want to stimulate your body's healing process without you needing to resort to medications and surgery. Though we are not against traditional medicine when it is required, we feel that many of these options may interfere with your natural healing abilities or simply cover up your symptoms temporarily.

Our Team

Our practice serves all ages and conditions.
Contact us today to get started.
cryonextintegrative.com/contact-us

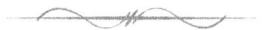

The Use of Modalities in Medicine

Modalities in medicine are different types of therapeutic approach.

We have several cutting-edge innovative recovery modalities in our clinic, including:

Chiropractic Care

Each of us is different, and the approach to health care should be unique, too. Our goal is to tailor each treatment to you. There are numerous techniques that Dr. Robert has mastered, including both manual and instrument-based methods.

Chiropractic care provides added benefits such as:

- increased energy
- decreased fatigue
- more restful sleep patterns
- decreased joint pains
- reduced stress
- mood enhancement
- increased focus

Whole Body Cryotherapy

Since the 1970s when cryotherapy was introduced to treat rheumatoid arthritis, its applications have skyrocketed. A quick, three-minute session causes a physiological response in the body that penetrates to your core. The blood moves from the extremities inward in an attempt to generate heat, where it is re-oxygenated and sent back to the extremities to stimulate the healing process. After a cryotherapy session, you will feel increased energy, mood enhancement, and increased focus. Whether you are an athlete in search of a superior recovery method, or someone looking to get rid of the chronic aches and pains, cryotherapy can help.

LED Light Therapy (Photobiomodulation)

LED light therapy or red light therapy stimulates healing in the body. This healing process continues well after the light is removed. There is substantial research to support the benefits of LED light therapy.

LED light plays a role in triggering healing, improving metabolism, increasing collagen production, restoring or promoting enzymes to speed the healing process, creating more ATP which means more energy, and increasing DNA synthesis. As a result, LED light therapy has been effective in treating aches and pains, arthritis, acne, wrinkles, inflammation, wounds and scars, anxiety and skin disorders.

At CryoNext Integrative Healthcare, you have access to the only full-body LED bed that combines LED light therapy and Nogier frequencies.

Fascial Stretch Therapy

Fascia is the body's connective tissue. It is the all-encompassing and interwoven system of fibrous connective tissue found throughout the body. The fascia provides a framework that helps to support and protect individual muscle groups, organs as well as the entire body.

Fascial Stretch Therapy is done on a massage table, using stabilizing straps to isolate one side at a time and provide support. The 60-minute full body session uses traction, the practitioner's' body weight as leverage, and modified PNF (client-assisted stretching) to increase range of motion and flexibility. It releases tension and breaks up the adhesions in the fascia, freeing up movement in the ligaments, tendons and muscles.

Fascial Stretch Therapy is gaining momentum as it has become an integral part of sports performance and recovery, as well as injury prevention, and has gained popularity with professional athletes around the world. Our therapists have treated numerous professional athletes including members of Orlando Magic, the Baltimore Orioles and professional boxers and MMA fighters.

Compression Therapy

NormaTec Pulse Massage Pattern employs three key techniques to enhance blood flow and maximize your recovery:

1. **Pulsing:** Instead of using static compression (squeezing) to transport fluid out of the limbs, Sequential Pulse Technology uses dynamic compression (pulsing). The pulsing action more effectively mimics the muscle pump of the legs and arms, greatly enhancing the

movement of fluid and metabolites out of the limbs after an intense workout.

2. **Gradients:** Veins and lymphatic vessels have one-way valves that prevent fluid backflow. Similarly, NormaTec Pulse Technology uses hold pressures to keep fluids from being forced in the wrong direction. Because of this enhancement, instead of tapering pressure off, the Pulse and Pulse Pro can deliver maximum pressure in every zone.

3. **Distal Release:** Because extended static pressure can be detrimental to the body's normal circulatory flow, Sequential Pulse Technology releases the hold pressures once they are no longer needed to prevent backflow. By releasing the hold pressure in each zone as soon as possible, each portion of the limb gains maximal rest time without a significant pause between compression cycles.

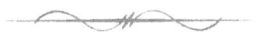

Who's to Blame for America's Health Crisis?

People tend to think of today's health crisis in the United States as a health *insurance* crisis. Fingers have been pointed at many parties for the current state of affairs:

- Government, for the lack of universal and affordable health insurance.
- Pharmaceutical companies, for the ever-increasing price of prescription drugs.
- Health care industry, for poor managed health care practices.
- Food industry, because lower income individuals are practically forced to purchase cheap, highly processed, unhealthy foods.

Although each of these parties has a hand in perpetuating the crisis, none of them is the true cause. The real reason behind the health care crisis is each individual's poor choices and lifestyle, mostly in the areas of food, exercise, and stress management. This leads to health-related issues like cancer, heart disease, metabolic syndrome, stroke, diabetes, and so much more.

Whether we like it or not, each one of us must take personal responsibility for our health. This means educating ourselves about the choices that will make a positive change for us and for those we love.

Biggest Health Issue Is Big Indeed

Perhaps the biggest health issue in the United States is obesity. In fact, it is at epidemic proportions. Among Americans age 20 and older, 154.7 million are overweight or obese.[1]

18% of deaths in America are associated with obesity. These deaths stem primarily from type 2 diabetes, hypertension, heart disease, liver disease, cancer, dementia, and depression.[2]

How Did the Obesity Problem Get So Big?

Early in the 20th century, the American diet was quite different from what it is today. If you could hop in a time machine and peek onto the shelves at the local store your grandparents shopped at, you would find produce, living plants, seeds, and grains. You might also find some home canned products. You would not find today's grocery store travesties:

- hormone injected meats
- processed foods
- fast foods
- junk foods

With these "modern" food choices comes a completely different diet – the SAD diet (Standard American Diet). The foods found in the SAD diet are completely out of balance.

1. an excessive amount of meat, fats, and sugar
2. too few fruits and vegetables

3. lack of nutrients in the food due to overcooking and processing

Incredibly, billions of dollars have been spent on various studies in a quest to find the causes and solutions for obesity. But the real answer is sitting in plain sight in homes across America: specifically, in the kitchens and on the couches.

The answer to the obesity crisis and the health care crisis in general is simple – return to a more natural diet rich in fresh fruits and vegetables, avoid processed foods, and be more active every day.

Trying to Make the Perfect Food Better

Food companies work tirelessly at making the perfect foods – fruits, vegetables and grains – better by refining them and processing them and adding chemicals to them. Ironically, all this tinkering has created an American diet that is deficient.

Processed foods make up a huge percentage of the American diet. These food products are loaded with extra salt, sugar, artificial flavors, preservatives, and other chemicals. These foods are also missing vital nutrients and vitamins that are stripped away during processing. This adding and subtracting from our food is a recipe for disaster.

Whole, natural foods are perfect foods. Eating a wide variety of fruits, vegetables, and grains gives your body everything it needs for good health. The SAD diet does not.

What It Is and What It Isn't

The Standard American Diet, sadly, is high in calories and low in nutrition. It consists of foods such as:

- refined flour
- refined sugar
- refined cooking oil
- soft drinks
- coffee
- margarine
- distilled liquor

In order to be healthy, we need to replace low nutrient foods with high nutrient, non-processed foods, including:

- vegetables
- fruits
- lean meat in moderation
- fish

A healthy body needs a diet high in vitamins, minerals, enzymes and antioxidants. It's the best way to make sure your body can correctly digest food, absorb nutrients, regulate cell function, and keep your body fueled up.

When your body doesn't have the nutrients it needs, the aging process speeds up. Aging doesn't just mean gray hair and wrinkles – we are talking about all the diseases associated with aging, such as:

- Coronary Heart Disease (CHD): About 600,000 people die of heart disease in the United States every year–that's 1 in every 4 deaths.[3]
- Coronary heart disease alone costs the United States $108.9 billion each year.[4]
- Stroke: In 2009, stroke caused 1 of every 19 deaths in the United States. On average, every 40 seconds,

someone in the United States has a stroke. Every four minutes, someone dies from a stroke.[5]

- High Blood Pressure: Based on data from 2007 to 2010, about 78 million people in the United States age 20 and older have high blood pressure.[6]

- Cancer: In 2012, there were approximately 13.7 million Americans with a history of cancer. Some of these men and women were cancer-free and others still had evidence of cancer and could be undergoing treatment. In 2013, there were expected to be 1,660,290 new cancer cases.[7]

- Diabetes: Data from the 2011 National Diabetes Fact Sheet states that 25.8 million people in the United States has diabetes. 1.9 million new adult cases of diabetes were diagnosed in 2010. An update in 2013 states that the total cost of diagnosed diabetes in the United States in 2012 was $245 billion.[8]

- Osteoporosis: More than 40 million Americans are estimated to already have this disease.[9]

The United States is reported to spend over eight thousand dollars per person on healthcare.[10] It is hard to believe that there are people dying of an inadequate diet in the United States when there is a surplus of food, but it's true. And there appears to be little hope of reversing the trend.

The World Health Organization (WHO) ranked the U.S. number one in health care spending. But even with all this spending, the U.S. ranked 72 in overall health – lower than many Third World countries.[11]

The Real Answer

People like to think that modern medicine is the answer to the health care crisis. But experts in the field of medicine realize that despite the use of advanced technology, there has been no decline in the health crisis.

The real answer does not rely on the curing of disease, but in the prevention of it. And one of the best ways to prevent disease is living a healthy lifestyle. For many people, understanding what constitutes a healthy lifestyle is daunting. Other people know exactly what "healthy living" means, but they are not willing to commit to making the necessary lifestyle changes. Committing to choices like these simply sounds like too much of a hassle:

1. Eat well – Kick the SAD diet out of your life and replace it with a diet filled with fresh fruits and vegetables, whole grains(limited), lean meats, healthy fats, and fish.
2. Exercise well – Exercising just 30 minutes three times per week will promote heart health, help you lose weight by increasing your metabolism, build strong bones, and boost your immune system.
3. Sleep well –Most cell repairs and memory assimilation happen during sleep. Most people need seven to eight hours of sleep each night in order to function at their best.
4. Live well – Believe it or not, kindness and love, as well as having a set of principles to guide your life, will help you to be healthier and live longer.
5. Optimal Nervous System Health – Everything that goes on in our body begins with the nervous system. Ridding your body of blockages in the nervous system, known as subluxation, can help you reach your full potential.

The burden of achieving good health falls squarely on your own shoulders. You cannot rely on others to watch out for your health. You cannot find good health at the doctor's office or in the pharmacy. You can't find it in the junk food aisles of the grocery store or in fast food restaurants. Good health can only be found when you commit to a healthy lifestyle.

By taking care of your body now, learning everything you can to make good choices, and finding practitioners that promote the prevention of disease, you will be well on your way to a healthier you.

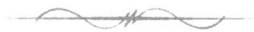

The Crisis Care Dilemma

Modern medicine is crisis-focused. It's one of the things that allows the average American to burn the candle at both ends for a few decades, have a little open heart surgery to keep the old ticker chugging along, and skid into a late retirement exhausted, disabled, and broke.

Think about it.

Are you motivated to be well right now, or will you be far more motivated to be well when you get sick and your life is taken away from you? Sadly, we only tend to find our motivation when something goes wrong. It's far easier to choose cheeseburgers and couch time over healthier choices... until all those bad choices finally create a disaster for our health.

That's the real cause of the vast majority of diseases we are dealing with today: lifestyle choices. We should be motivated every day to live a lifestyle that allows us to thrive, maintain, and enjoy a fantastic quality of life. And that's what the wellness movement is all about: seeking wellness instead of seeking cures, each and every day. There is no medication, special lotion, injection or surgery that will magically restore your health.

Modern medicine runs on the philosophy that aging is the decline phase of life. We are born, we live, we get sick, and we die. But it doesn't have to be that way! There's the first mindset switch we need to make. Instead of thinking of our bodies as vessels destined and designed for deterioration and disease, think of it as being meant for continuous progress. Yes, we will all age, and we will all eventually die. But how would the rest of your life be different if you decided to live up to your physical potential from here on out?

What Is Wellness Care?

More and more people are coming to realize that focusing on their wellness could allow them to live healthier, longer lives. They are demanding that their health care providers work with them on wellness plans that prevent, rather than cure, diseases and pain. There is evidence of this shift all around us:

- Organic and local foods are becoming the preferred produce option in America, and around the world. The USDA's National Farmers Market Directory's listings have increased by more than 61% since 2008.[12]
- The Veterans Administration has committed to implementing alternative therapies to help veterans deal with pain and avoid possible opioid painkiller addictions.[13]
- According to Harvard Medical School, Americans make about 425 million visits to holistic health care providers each year.[14]
- A 2011 Gallup poll showed that half of Americans take vitamins every day.[15]

Part of the wellness revolution has been a shift in the relationship between primary care doctors and patients. By and large, the public no longer chooses to take their doctor's advice as the final word on certain health concerns. We are far more likely today to ask questions, seek second opinions, and research alternative treatments. The patient, rather than the doctor, is now the decision-maker when the patient's wellness is concerned.

What IS Modern Medicine Good For?

Make no mistake: modern medicine still plays an important role in our health care system. And the more open and receptive your primary care physician is to discuss your wellness care, the more of a partner role he or she can play in your ongoing health.

The modern view on health care places all health-related concepts and activities into three categories:

1. Self Care – this includes the choices you make every day about diet, exercise, stress management, and so on.
2. Health Care – this is all of the things you seek help for to maintain good health, such as seeking wellness providers, getting educated on fitness and exercise, and taking part in wellness programs physicians are offering.
3. Crisis Care – this is the care we obtain when a disaster strikes. When we get sick or injured, we go to the doctor to help us fix what we cannot handle on our own.

Self care and health care are intended to prevent the need for crisis care. However, choosing to stop smoking will not prevent you from getting into a car accident. There are sure-fire ways to prevent cancer, heart attacks, or other conditions, but of course there are occurrences were serious illnesses, broken bones, failing organs - situations such as these are the rightful domain of crisis care.

A Crash Course in How to Get Well

America's current health care system promotes drugs and surgery above all else – including prevention. Each year, America spends $3 billion on prescription medications and $2 trillion on crisis care.[16] The first tragedy of this situation is that despite all that spending, America is still getting sicker and sicker. The second tragedy is that most of the illnesses for which we seek crisis care are completely preventable.

There are about a hundred lifestyle choices you could improve upon. Here are a few simple suggestions to get you back on track:

- Get regular, moderate exercise
- Stay well hydrated
- Eat a plant-based, nutrient-dense diet
- Get adequate sleep
- Quit smoking and any other drug habits
- Enjoy moderate alcohol intake at the most
- Find healthy ways to deal with stress
- Seek activities and people that boost your mood
- Bring aboard health care practitioners you trust to help you feel well

In later chapters, we will dig into many of these topics in more detail. Suffice it to say that people tend to feel stressed and conflicted when making these lifestyle shifts. It's just so much easier to give in to our desires... to be lazy and not hit the gym... to order the cheeseburger because it's on the happy hour menu but the salad isn't... to quit smoking, maybe next week.

All of those choices we make every day seem insignificant in the moment. But it all adds up. In ten, twenty, thirty years from now, will you regret your lifestyle choices? What it all comes down to is this – how can you improve your current level of functioning?

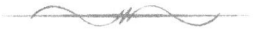

What You Need to Know about Peripheral Neuropathy

What is Peripheral Neuropathy? It helps to break the term down and look at each individual word. **Neuropathy** refers to pain that is caused by nerve damage. The **peripheral** part of the term refers to the peripheral nervous system – that's all of the nerves in your body that radiate out from your spinal cord. So peripheral neuropathy is typically presented as pain and tingling caused by nerve damage in the extremities.

The most common areas affected by peripheral neuropathy are the nerves in the extremities, like your arms, hands, legs, and feet. People with peripheral neuropathy generally describe the pain as stabbing, tingling, numbness, burning, or icy coldness. Many of these patients also report some weakness in the affected area.

Neuropathy of the small fiber nerves reduces sensation and can cause the patient not to be able to feel cuts, burns, punctures, or blisters on the skin. Reduced sensation in the feet can cause car accidents when people fail to sense whether they are pressing the gas pedal or the brake, or they may not be able to regulate the pressure they apply to a pedal.

Neuropathy of the large fiber nerves in the legs can cause loss of balance and coordination. This type of neuropathy causes thousands of falls every year. A fall puts the patient at risk for hip fractures, head traumas, and other serious injuries.

In addition to the extremities, other parts of the body can be affected by neuropathy; for example, the peripheral nervous system also controls your vital organs. Damage to the associated nerves can cause heartburn, indigestion, difficulty swallowing, constipation, and many other problems.

What Causes Peripheral Neuropathy?

Instead of delving into the hundreds of specific causes there are for peripheral neuropathy, we will break them down into three general categories.

1. **Circulation related peripheral neuropathy** is most often experienced by people with diabetes, but anyone with reduced blood circulation is at risk. When the small blood vessels surrounding the nerves die off, the nerves are deprived of nourishment and will also eventually die. The damaged nerves are the source of the pain and tingling.

    Over 50% of diabetics develop some form of neuropathy (Mayo Clinic). Peripheral neuropathy is also the top cause of amputations for diabetics.

2. **Toxicity related peripheral neuropathy** can be caused by any sort of exposure to toxins. The two causes we typically focus on are chemotherapy drugs and statins.

    a. **Chemotherapy-induced peripheral neuropathy** is a side effect reported by many cancer patients. Some chemotherapy drugs are more likely to cause neuropathy than others. Patients who are on a more frequent treatment schedule are also more likely to experience neuropathy.

    b.   **Statin-induced peripheral neuropathy** is caused by the use of drugs that doctors prescribe to reduce fats, including triglycerides and cholesterol, in the blood. Instead of prescribing changes in diet and exercise habits to fix the root cause of the cholesterol problem, it is far easier (and more profitable) for a doctor to prescribe a statin.

3.   **Trauma induced peripheral neuropathy** is caused by events like car accidents, falls, or athletic injuries. Any of these events can cause damage to the peripheral nerves. Wearing a cast, walking with crutches, or frequent repetitive motions can also damage nerves. (Mayo Clinic)

One important fact to realize is that regardless of the cause of peripheral neuropathy, the damage is the same under a microscope. The techniques for rebuilding the nerves do not change.

How Do You Treat Peripheral Neuropathy?

Medical doctors routinely tell their patients that nerves cannot regenerate themselves, but it's simply not true! Several treatments have been proven to stimulate the growth of the nerve endings and the blood vessels that nourish them.

If the symptoms are caused by a treatable underlying condition, it is almost always possible to reverse the neuropathy. While medications can reduce the pain associated with peripheral neuropathy, painkillers do nothing to repair or reverse the damage to the nerves and blood vessels. Getting to the root cause of the neuropathy and taking steps to reverse the damage is the only effective and long-lasting method of treatment.

The end goal in treating peripheral neuropathy is to remove blockage so that the nerves can function properly and send and receive messages with the brain. The best way to achieve this is with a comprehensive treatment plan. That's why we use several methods concurrently to treat our peripheral neuropathy patients. At our clinic, peripheral neuropathy appointments last about 45 minutes rather than the standard 15-minute visit.

Peripheral Neuropathy Treatment Options

Low Level Light Therapy (LLLT) – LLLT uses low-power lasers or infrared light-emitting diodes to promote nerve growth, reduce pain, improve immune response, accelerate healing of wounds and fractures, increase collagen and DNA production, and promote fibroblast activity.

Vibration Therapy – Vibration therapy increases balance and mobility, bone density, and range of motion. It also increases blood flow by 15 times. During vibration therapy, patients sit or stand on a vibrating platform that causes their muscles to contract, increase circulation, as well as nerve stimulation.

ReBuilder System – Uses electrical stimulation of the muscles to improve blood flow and normalize deficits in nerve conduction velocity. The ReBuilder System is trusted by all four Cancer Treatment Centers of America locations to alleviate chemotherapy-induced peripheral neuropathy. Most of their cancer patients who use the Re-Builder System have reduced or stopped taking their pain medicine, as they report drastically reduced pain in their extremities after treatments.

Soft Tissue Therapy-Hand-held soft tissue machines are used to massage the tissue surrounding the areas affected by peripheral neuropathy. Soft tissue therapy targets injured muscles and soft tissue. Massage, pressure, stretching and trigger point techniques are used to promote the restoration of function, improved circulation, and breaking down scar tissue.

Spinal Decompression - When peripheral neuropathy has resulted from an accident or injury that resulted in compressed discs or vertebrae, spinal decompression can provide relief. Spinal decompression is a chiropractic technique that uses traction to take the pressure off the discs and allow the discs to move back into place. It also stimulates blood flow, which produces a healing response.

Traditional chiropractic therapy is used by millions of people to adjust misaligned vertebrae. Regular chiropractic care allows signals to flow between the brain, spinal cord, and nerves. Since chiropractic adjustments promote nervous system function, it should be considered an integral part of any peripheral neuropathy treatment plan. More importantly, chiropractic is used to get the feet and hands more mobile as the neuropathy creates stiffness and mobility problems.

Each intricate part of our program is equally important. Each one relies on the other to do its job. There are a lot of treatments out there that get new blood to the areas temporarily. We know them all; our goal is to repair neuropathy permanently.

These treatment methods will be discussed in more detail in the following chapters.

What Else Can I Do to Reduce My Pain?

There are additional components of a full peripheral neuropathy treatment plan that cannot be controlled in the clinic setting. While we provide our patients with the resources to make the right choices for themselves, it is solely up to them how closely they follow these guidelines.

Nutrition – Committing to dietary changes that reduce inflammation in the body can make a tremendous difference in peripheral neuropathy symptoms. Basically, an anti-inflammatory diet promotes foods that inhibit inflammation (fruits, vegetables, lean omega-3 rich foods) and limits the intake of foods that promote inflammation (sugars, starches, omega-6 foods).

Supplements – Natural Nitric Oxide Boosters is an intricate part of for treating peripheral neuropathy. In the following chapters, we will take a closer look at the peripheral neuropathy treatment options we offer in our clinic.

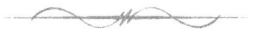

Low Level Light Therapy (Photobiomodulation)

Since lasers were invented in the 1960's, medical professionals have discovered numerous applications for lasers to improve people's health. Ophthalmologists, dermatologists, and surgeons quickly found lasers to be useful in treating their patients. Low level light therapy (LLLT) or photobiomodulation is in its fourth decade of use as a method of treating sprains, back and neck pain, arthritis, ulcers, and more.

Looking to the future, studies are currently being conducted to test out LLLT's effectiveness in treating sperm mobility, spinal cord injuries, stroke victims, Parkinson's patients, and Alzheimer's disease.

How Does LLLT Work?

Think back to your high school biology class. You may recall that plants use a process called photosynthesis to produce energy. The plant changes that energy into ATP, which is the fuel stored and used by all cells in all living things – plants and animals alike. LLLT stimulates the production of enzyme cytochrome c oxidase, which, like sunlight for plants, produces ATP. With more fuel being produced, cells have more energy to repair themselves. Currently, numerous studies being conducted around the world are proving that LLLT can help the body regenerate its own tissues, including spinal cord and nerve tissues. The therapy also holds promise for restoring eyesight, reversing numerous neurological diseases, and stroke recovery.

What Else Could LLLT Treat in the Future?

Fibromyalgia is a condition that causes the brain to process pain abnormally, resulting in chronic, widespread pain and chronic fatigue. This condition affects millions of Americans and has been poorly understood and underdiagnosed, resulting in billions of dollars in cost to our health care system.

Fibromyalgia is primarily treated with medications; side effects often make the patient's symptoms even worse. But studies have already shown that LLLT helps to treat the pain and swelling of fibromyalgia.

Parkinson's disease is caused by the loss of dopamine-producing brain cells. The four primary symptoms of Parkinson's disease are tremors in the arms, legs, jaw, and face; stiffness of the limbs and trunk; slowness of movement; and impaired balance and coordination.

Many scientists think that one of the malfunctioning systems in Parkinson's disease is located in the mitochondria. These are the cellular systems/organelles that produce ATP, the energy for all the other systems of the body. They also help to detoxify the brain and body by regulating the free radicals circulating in the system.

A study by the UVA Morris K. Udall Parkinson's Research Center of Excellence showed that a single, brief treatment of LLLT increased the movement of the mitochondria in neuron cells to be similar to the level of movement in disease-free, age-matched control groups.[17]

Muscle regeneration is another area where LLLT holds great promise. LLLT has been shown to increase cellular function and regeneration, including cells that create muscle tissue. Studies are being conducted to determine if heart muscles can be regenerated using LLLT.

Medical doctors are taught that heart muscle does not regenerate. Therefore, when someone has a heart attack, doctors tell patients that the muscle that died in the attack is gone for good. However, new research shows that heart muscle can and does regenerate. This finding opens up new possibilities of regenerating heart muscle after a heart attack with LLLT, thereby preventing a host of complications including heart failure.

Weight loss might sound like a stretch when you think of the possibilities of LLLT treatment, but it is already being used to help patients achieve their goals. Laser light easily penetrates through layers of skin to activate healing responses within cells and to stimulate nerve endings to produce endorphins. Endorphins, such as serotonin, are produced normally by your body and are nature's natural mood lifter and help prevent you from feeling anxious or moody.

The LLLT therapy of specific points on the body helps to reduce the desire to eat, providing a natural satiation without food. The laser also helps balance organ and glandular functions that regulate weight. Incredibly, LLLT is used in a very similar way to relieve the withdrawal symptoms of quitting smoking!

Diabetic ulcers are one of the many health risks associated with uncontrolled diabetes. Diabetic ulcers are extremely hard to cure. Due to artery abnormalities, diabetic neuropathy, and delayed wound healing, infection or gangrene of the extremities is relatively common.

Wound healing is usually taken care of efficiently by a healthy body. But diabetes is a disorder that impedes normal steps of the wound healing process. Common treatments - skin grafts, moist wound therapy, and negative pressure wound therapy – almost never work completely.

LLLT is a new treatment option for diabetic ulcers that is showing great promise. Unlike other therapies, LLLT has no side effects. In one case study, a man with a diabetic ulcer was treated for a total of 16 sessions of low-intensity laser therapy over a four-week period. During this time, the ulcer healed completely. During a follow-up period of nine months, there was no recurrence of the ulcer.[18]

Skin disorders: LLLT appears to have a wide range of application in dermatology, especially in conditions where stimulation of healing, reduction of inflammation, reduction of cell death and skin rejuvenation are required. The application of LLLT to pigmentation disorders may work both ways by producing both repigmentation of vitiligo, and depigmentation of hyperpigmented lesions depending on the dose.[19]

What Role Does LLLT Play in Treating Peripheral Neuropathy?

Because LLLT stimulates cellular regeneration, it plays a vital role in a complete treatment plan for peripheral neuropathy patients. LLLT helps damaged nerves and their surrounding blood vessels regrow, gradually improving sensation and function for the patient. There are currently no drugs on the market that can help the body heal itself in such a way. Plus, unlike virtually all medications, there are absolutely no side effects associated with LLLT. The area may feel warm or tingly during the treatment, but there are no other reported physical sensations from LLLT patients.

When a patient visits our office for treatment of peripheral neuropathy, we apply LLLT boots around the hands, feet, or both and let the machine deliver the treatment for a specified amount of time.

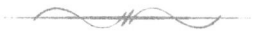

Electrotherapy for Pain Relief and Nerve Re-education

Right off the bat, let's get one thing out of the way: this is nothing like the horrifying practice of electroshock therapy that was used in asylums decades ago. And on the other hand, it's more exciting than the electrolysis procedure that can get rid of unwanted body hair.

Electrotherapy is a pain management technique where small electrical currents stimulate nerves and muscles to release pain-killing chemicals such as endorphins, and prevents pain signals from being transmitted to the brain. Electrotherapy also improves nerve function by gently opening up the nerve pathways. It does not hurt your muscles or nerves, and it does not burn your skin. In our office, we rely on the ReBuilder System for patients seeking treatment for peripheral neuropathy. This technology is much different than a TENS unit. TENS units can actually make neuropathy worse over time.

ReBuilder is an FDA-approved device that was designed specifically to treat the pain, burning, numbness, and tingling associated with peripheral neuropathy. In fact, all of the Cancer Treatment Centers of America use Rebuilder to alleviate the chemotherapy-induced neuropathy of their patients.

What Are the Benefits of ReBuilder Treatment?

Daily, thirty-minute ReBuilder treatments in your home may significantly reduce the amount of pain medications needed to deal with an acute pain syndrome. It has also been used to effectively treat functional problems such as drop foot. The effects of this treatment method are cumulative, meaning that the longer you continue to use it, the better the results you will see.

ReBuilder also increases blood flow, strengthens muscles, and improves the transmission of signals within the nervous system. And when patients experience less pain at night, they tend to get a better night's sleep. This allows them to function better during the daytime and promotes cellular repair and regeneration during their restful hours.

How Do I Use ReBuilder at Home?

You will place small adhesive pads in a supplied footbath, or place the affected areas on specific pads in order to deliver electrical current. Your healthcare provider will help you determine where the pads should be placed for best results. The vast majority of patients, marked improvement in pain, function, and mobility occurs within just a few electrotherapy treatments.

How does it work?

All you have to do is put on the pads or garments, turn on the system, and sit back so that the device can do its job. ReBuilder is an "intelligent" system, in that it analyzes the nerves 7.83 times per second, determines the correct amount of electrical signal, and then delivers it to the target area.[20]

The electrical current opens up the nerve pathways and promotes good signal conduction. During treatment, you may feel your muscles contract and relax – this is normal. As you progress through more and more treatments, your condition will improve and the need for electrotherapy is reduced. Throughout the treatment period, the ReBuilder will alter the amount of signal it delivers based on the condition of your nerves.

Whether your peripheral neuropathy is a side effect of statin drugs, chemotherapy treatment, diabetes, or another source, ReBuilder can help restore function and sensation to your peripheral nervous system.

Why Is ReBuilder the Electrotherapy System of Choice?

Since ReBuilder hit the market in the mid 1980's, it has helped millions of patients repair their pain points from the inside out with no drugs, no surgery, and virtually no side effects. When you have dealt with problems like shortness of breath, memory loss, constipation, sleeplessness, and dizziness while on pain medications, the idea of treating the root cause of the pain and eliminating drugs from your daily routine often seems like nothing more than a fantasy. But it's totally possible – perhaps within a week or two – with electrotherapy.

Another benefit of the ReBuilder System is that it shuts off automatically when the treatment time is up. This prevents possible injury, should the patient fall asleep during treatment. ReBuilder also comes with a lifetime warranty.

But the real reason we use ReBuilder for our peripheral neuropathy patients is simple: we have seen the results first-hand. Almost all of our patients who use ReBuilder report feeling less numbness, pain, and tingling in the treated area. With blood flow and nerve function restored, patients become more mobile and stop relying on painkillers to get through the day.

Is ReBuilder Right for Me?

In our clinic, we are all about helping our patients heal from the inside out, without medications or surgery. We use several modalities at once to treat our patients who are suffering from peripheral neuropathy because we believe in a broad-spectrum approach to treating chronic pain. All of the techniques we combine for neuropathy treatment are focused on improving nerve function and regeneration, as well as promoting blood flow.

Our neuropathy patients come to us in the midst of a very difficult period in their lives. They may be going through chemotherapy treatment; maybe they are failing to recover from an automobile accident; they could also be suffering from diabetes-induced neuropathy. While the causes of their pain are different, we use similar methods to treat them all. Electrotherapy is one important treatment method that they all have in common.

Thousands of doctors in all types of practices prescribe the ReBuilder System for their patients. All four Cancer Treatment Centers of America offer it to their patients who are undergoing chemotherapy. And as a matter of fact, using Rebuilder *before* starting treatment can be an effective preventative measure against developing peripheral neuropathy in the first place.[21]

If you are suffering from the effects of peripheral neuropathy, there is an excellent chance that ReBuilder can help. The ReBuilder is only a piece of the puzzle in our innovative program. We strongly believe that a more complete approach to neuropathy reversal is a smarter plan of action. That's why we prescribe electrotherapy, low level light therapy, chiropractic, nutrition, and vibration therapy to our patients who are struggling to get their pain under control and live an active life like they desire.

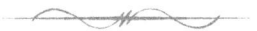

Soft Tissue Therapy
That Keeps You Moving

Soft tissue therapy includes a variety of massage-type treatments of the soft tissue, which includes muscles, connective tissue, ligaments, and tendons. Soft tissue therapy can effectively treat injuries, pain, and dysfunction.

Soft tissue therapy can help with:

- Carpal tunnel syndrome
- Joint pain
- Shin splints
- Back pain
- Plantar fasciitis
- Fibromyalgia
- Tendinitis
- Groin pulls
- Frozen shoulder

Benefits of Soft Tissue Therapy

Soft tissue therapy is effective in alleviating many symptoms associated with those medical conditions listed above. It can improve the performance of your muscles, circulatory system, joints and immune system. For better range of motion, decreased blood pressure, and to alleviate the pain and stiffness associated with arthritis or fibromyalgia, soft tissue therapy is the drug-free answer you're looking for.

Types of Soft Tissue Therapy

While some soft tissue therapies are delivered by chiropractors, others are offered by massage therapists.

Trigger Point Therapy

Trigger points are those tender "knots" you feel when you or someone rubs a sore spot. Your chiropractor will apply pressure to trigger points to relieve pain and dysfunction in other parts of the body – this is called trigger point therapy.

There are two basic types of trigger points: active and latent.

- Active trigger points cause muscular pain and transfer pain to other areas of the body when your chiropractor applies pressure. For example, pressing on a trigger point between your shoulders may send shooting pain down your arm.
- Latent trigger points do not refer pain to other areas of the body, and cause stiffness in the joints and restricted range of motion.

Trigger points develop due to several causes, including birth trauma, an injury sustained in a fall or accident, poor posture, or overexertion.

After several treatments of trigger point therapy, the swelling and stiffness of muscular pain is reduced, range of motion is increased, tension is relieved, and circulation, flexibility and coordination are improved.

Swedish massage

Swedish massage is the most common type of massage in the United States. In Swedish massage, your massage therapist will lubricate the skin with massage oil and use various strokes, like gliding, kneading, friction, stretching and tapping, to warm up and work the muscle tissue. This helps to release tension and break up muscle knots. This mode of treatment helps to reduce swelling and inflammation, as well as promote relaxation.

Cross-Friction massage

Soft tissues can become stressed beyond their limits, resulting in small, microscopic tears. When these tears occur, the body responds by causing inflammation, which helps in the role of healing. However, too much inflammation can form scar tissue.

Continuing to use the muscle as it is torn can increase the chance of more scarring. Scar tissue is tough and decreases mobility and elasticity. This results in loss of function, resulting in more tearing and inflammation, resulting in more scar tissue... a vicious cycle.

For cross friction massage, your massage therapist will apply his fingers directly over the tissue involved. The key here is for the massage to be opposite the direction of the tissue fibers. This "transverse friction" massage keeps adhesions and scar tissue from forming. It also results in improved range of motion and less pain.

Cross friction massage is a highly effective treatment for injuries to the muscles, tendons, and ligaments caused by micro-tears. Cross friction creates heat, which helps to mobilize adhesions (bands of scar tissue) between fascial layers, muscles, and other soft tissues. This heat helps to promote healing.

Knee injuries are extremely common, but the healing process can be quite frustrating. In a 2009 study, bilateral knee injuries were treated with cross friction massage one week following injury. Fifty-one participants received between nine and 30 treatments. After four weeks of cross friction massage, the knees were stronger, less stiff and could absorb more energy.[22]

Myofascial release therapy

Myofascial release is a stretching technique used by chiropractors to treat soft tissue problems. To understand what it is and how it works, you first need to know a few things about fascia.

Fascia is a thin tissue that covers the muscles and every fiber within each muscle. This means that when you stretch your muscles, you are really stretching your muscles and your fascia.

When muscle fibers are injured, the fibers and the fascia surrounding it become short and tight. This uneven stress can cause pain and other symptoms. Myofascial release treats these symptoms by releasing the uneven tightness in injured fascia.

The stretching is determined by your chiropractor as he feels what each stretch does to your body. The feedback he receives helps him decide how much force to use, the direction of the stretch, and how long to stretch.

Your chiropractor will find areas of tightness and then apply a light stretch. Once your muscle and fascia have relaxed, he will increase the stretch. This process is repeated until the area is fully relaxed. Then, the next affected area is stretched.

One area that myofascial release therapy holds great promise is in the treatment of scoliosis, which is an abnormal curvature of the spine. A 2008 case study of an 18-year-old female subject observed her progress as she underwent six weeks of myofascial release therapy. The subject received treatment consisting of two sessions each week for 60 minutes. Pain, pulmonary function and quality of life were measured at predetermined intervals. The subject improved with pain levels, trunk rotation, posture, quality of life, and pulmonary function.[23]

Active Release Therapy (ART)

One goal of Active Release Therapy (ART) is to restore normal texture, motion, and function of soft tissues. Another goal is to release any trapped nerves or blood vessels. This is accomplished through the removal of adhesions as your chiropractor applies stretching and massage techniques.

Adhesions happen for two reasons. One reason is acute injury, such as a blow, fall, pull, or strain. The second reason is repetitive overuse, which can happen with improper posture, compensating for injuries (i.e. limping), or repetitive motions. The result is that the area is compressed and tissues suffer from decreased blood supply. The soft tissues respond by forming scar tissue. This results in pain, poor mobility, and a continued injury cycle.

Your chiropractor will determine which soft tissue is affected. Then specific massage techniques are used to make these tissues slide over one another with a hand, finger, or thumb.

In the first three levels of ART treatment, all movement is facilitated by your chiropractor. In level four of the treatment, your chiropractor will have you move in specific ways as he applies pressure.

ART is a great treatment option for carpal tunnel syndrome, sciatica, TMJ, and other problems.

Muscle Energy Technique (MET)

Muscle energy technique (MET) is based on the idea that muscles on one side of a joint relax as the other side of the joint contracts.

MET is used to:

- Lengthen shortened or spastic muscles
- Improve weakened ligaments and muscle strength
- Improve range of motion

During an MET treatment, your chiropractor will ask you to contract a muscle for approximately five seconds while he applies an anti-force to that muscle. Each time you contract your muscle, it stretches further. Muscle energy techniques can be applied safely to almost any joint in the body.

Graston Technique therapy

It helps your chiropractor break up scar tissue by the use of specially designed instruments to identify and treat areas exhibiting soft tissue issues. The edges of the tools mold to the various shapes of the body.

Graston Technique instruments act like tuning forks, vibrating in your chiropractor's hand. This allows him to find specific adhesions and restrictions and treat them precisely. Deeper adhesions can be better treated with Graston tools than without them.

Which type of soft tissue therapy is right for you?

Our team will evaluate what type of muscle work you may need. They will administer the appropriate treatments available when you go in for your evaluation. These treatments often work together to provide better circulation, pain relief and range of motion in a shorter amount of time than either modality can deliver on its own.

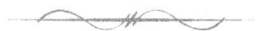

Surprising Relief Comes from Vibration Therapy

Healthcare providers, physical therapists, chiropractors, and personal trainers use whole-body vibration therapy (WBVT) for a surprisingly wide range of conditions. Specifically, vibration therapy is great for:

- Increasing muscle endurance, coordination, and strength
- Better circulation of lymph fluid and blood for better healing, energy, and overall health
- Improving nerve activity
- Boosting bone density and fighting off osteoporosis

For our patients with peripheral neuropathy, vibration therapy reduces their pain, increases circulation, improves strength and flexibility, and increases energy, mobility, and balance. We achieve these results without drugs or invasive surgery.

A recent study showed that patients with diabetic peripheral neuropathy (DPN) specifically have much to gain from vibration therapy. Study participants were observed to determine how effective whole body vibration therapy really is in treating pain associated with DPN. The study's participants received three whole body vibration treatments per week for a month. Each session consisted of four rounds of three minutes of vibration. The study's results demonstrated significant pain reduction overall, and no side-effects were observed during the study.[24]

WBVT allows individuals to experience less pain without invasive surgery, and usually reduces or even eliminates the need for pain medication. The high-frequency vertical vibrations produced by the device assist in increasing circulation, rebuilding muscle tissue, improving range of motion, and reducing pain and stress. But the benefits go even further beyond getting off pain medications. Patients are likely to see far fewer serious injuries and infections due to increased sensation and better coordination. And diabetics in particular will be at lower risk of limb amputation due to reduced infection rates.

How does WBVT work?

Vibration therapy devices come in a range of forms. There are vibrating foot platforms that treat just peripheral neuropathy of the feet. Some practitioners use hand-held devices to target very specific areas of the body and fully customize the length and duration of treatment. Other health care providers prefer vibrating chairs or platforms that patients may sit or stand on for a full-body treatment. Either way, the high frequency vibration is an effective and safe treatment for the area(s) of the body affected by neuropathy.

Vibration therapy stimulates a patient's muscles to rapidly contract. Frequent tightening of a muscle will build and strengthen the muscle tissue, even when it's performed for small bits of time. As the muscle builds, its need for blood also grows. This is what stimulates blood vessels to grow and keep fueling the muscles with the nutrients they need during and after vibration therapy.

It's important to note that while traditional exercise is difficult and often uncomfortable for many patients dealing with chronic pain, vibration therapy cuts these complications out of the equation. When people have reduced sensation in their feet and hands, it can be downright dangerous to pick up free weights or hop onto a treadmill. But vibration therapy allows the patient to sit down throughout the "workout," even though muscles are being strengthened the entire time.

When the muscles are pushed and exerted in specific ways, the nerves can be stimulated to regrow their neural pathways and even repair or rebuild the damaged nerves.

An added bonus of vibration therapy is that it stimulates the release of osteoblasts from the nuclei in bone cells. Osteoblasts are what make it possible for bones to grow stronger by creating new bone cells.

All of these facts combined means that vibration therapy patients will regain sensation, strength, and stamina. Over time, the little things in life that used to be exhausting will become far easier. Eventually, patients get back to more normal routines and introduce regular moderate exercise to their daily calendars. It is truly an eye-opening experience to lose full use of parts of your body, and then gain it back again. Your priorities and your perspective will never be the same.

Is There Anybody Who Should NOT Experience WBVT?

Certain patients should not participate in vibration therapy, including patients with epilepsy, severe vertigo, or a detached retina. Also, if you are pregnant, vibration therapy is probably not safe for you.

For the rest of our patients who may benefit from it, we recommend vibration therapy, which we also provide in our office. Vibration therapy treatments usually last no more than about 15 minutes. But the key to effectively treating many conditions, including peripheral neuropathy, is to approach it with several different modalities. That's why we never treat a PN patient with just vibration therapy.

Our peripheral neuropathy patients commonly experience vibration therapy, low-level light therapy, soft tissue treatments, electrical stimulation, and a chiropractic adjustment during their visits. We treat these pain-related conditions with everything we've got because patient health, comfort, and satisfaction are paramount. We know that this multi-pronged approach is the best way to get people off painkillers and back on their feet.

That's why we also continuously counsel our patients about the importance of proper hydration and diet. You really are what you eat, so it's crucial to fuel your body with healthy, high-quality foods that will promote growth, healing, and wellness in every cell of your body.

Continue on to the next chapter to learn more about the role good nutrition plays in your recovery from peripheral neuropathy.

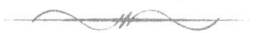

Good Health Starts with Good Nutrition

Getting regular exercise, dealing with stress in healthy ways, and eating a diet rich in plant-based whole foods is a great start toward achieving good health. But no matter how well you stick to these tips, you are always at risk for your body to be damaged at the cellular level. Environmental factors play a huge part in this damage by introducing free radicals into our bodies.

What Are Free Radicals?

Free radicals form in the human body when an electron in an atom becomes unpaired and searches for another electron to pair with. It may sounds like an insignificant event, but this search for another unpaired atom causes damage to our cells and a chain reaction of more free radical creation.

Daily life exposes us to free radicals all the time, from the foods we eat and the air we breathe. Free radicals cause illness and contribute to the aging process. They have a negative impact on how we look and feel. Free radicals occur in everyday life but are made worse by:

- eating a diet full of processed foods and produce treated with chemicals
- smoking
- pollution
- using drugs
- failure to deal correctly with stress
- excessive sun exposure

Free radical damage can lead to:

- cancer
- heart disease
- diabetes
- arthritis
- autoimmune diseases

One thing we can do to fight free radicals is to get more antioxidants in our diets. Antioxidants are vitamins, minerals, and other nutrients that protect the body and fight off free radicals. They give free radicals an electron to pair with before the stray electrons can damage our cells. Some examples of antioxidants are beta carotene, vitamin C, and vitamin E. These vitamins help strengthen the immune system, too. Plus, they're readily available in many plant-based foods which we should consume more of, anyway!

Beta Carotene

Beta carotene is one of a group of red, orange, and yellow pigments called carotenoids. Beta carotene and other carotenoids provide approximately 50% of the Vitamin A needed in our daily diet.[25]

Beta carotene is a substance the body converts into Vitamin A. It's a powerful antioxidant that also helps protect the cells and boost the immune system. Sources of this important nutrient include:

- carrots
- pumpkins
- sweet potatoes
- spinach
- collards
- kale
- turnip greens
- beet greens
- winter squash
- cabbage

If you would rather get your vitamin A straight-up instead of through the beta carotene conversion, eat more:

- broccoli
- cantaloupe
- apricots
- milk
- butter
- liver
- beef
- cheese
- whole eggs

Vitamin C

When your mom told you to drink orange juice to get over a cold faster, she was right! Vitamin C is another antioxidant that strengthens the immune system. It's vital to the growth and repair of skin, blood vessels, ligaments, and tendons. It is also involved with healing wounds and forming scar tissue.

Plus, vitamin C is important for the formation of collagen, which holds your body's cells together. And, it plays an important role in maintaining oral and eye health.

Many fruits are excellent sources of vitamin C, including:

- cantaloupe
- citrus fruits
- kiwi
- mango
- guava
- papaya
- pineapple
- berries
- watermelon

You can get vitamin C from vegetables too, like cruciferous veggies (broccoli, cauliflower, and Brussels sprouts), peppers, leafy greens, potatoes, tomatoes, and squash.

Vitamin E

The third antioxidant we're concerned about is vitamin E. This nutrient helps widen blood vessels and keeps blood from clotting inside them. Foods that are high in vitamin E will also protect your skin from ultraviolet light, which is a major cause of free radical formation in the body.

Excellent sources of vitamin E include:

- spinach
- chard
- turnip greens
- mustard greens
- cayenne pepper
- asparagus
- bell peppers
- olive oil
- whole grains
- nuts and seeds
- eggs
- meats

Nutrition

Eating a well-balanced diet should provide essential nutrients, but there are some situations that definitely call for adding in supplements. When your diet isn't properly balanced, it doesn't contain adequate amounts of certain nutrients. In this case, supplements may be absolutely necessary.

In order for our body to use food to repair and create cells and tissues, it needs the proper tools. The following nutrients are extremely important to maintain a healthy body. And just like the majority of antioxidant sources, these nutrients are often found in abundance in plant-sourced foods.

Magnesium is not only an essential nutrient but is responsible for a vast variety of healthy body functions. It also is the most deficient mineral in the Standard American Diet because it can be difficult to meet the daily requirements just from food. Less than 30% of U.S. adults consume the

Recommended Daily Allowance of magnesium. And nearly 20% get only half of the magnesium they need daily to remain healthy.[26]

To make sure you get enough magnesium in your diet, eat plenty of whole grains, legumes, vegetables, nuts, seeds, and seafood.

Calcium is the most abundant mineral in your body. It is responsible for strong teeth and bones, as well as proper function of blood vessels, nerve communication, and muscles. Many Americans suffer from a deficiency in calcium. We lose calcium each day through our skin, nails, hair, sweat, and waste.

To make sure you get enough calcium in your diet, make sure you consume dairy products, broccoli, kale, Chinese cabbage, and salmon regularly. Depending on your diet and age, your doctor might recommend a calcium supplement.

Iron is important for the production of hemoglobin (found in red blood cells) and myoglobin (found in muscles). These proteins carry and store oxygen throughout the body. When you don't have enough iron in your body you feel tired, weak, and unable to focus. Few people ever have too much iron in the body but this rare condition is toxic.

Excellent sources of iron include red meat, liver, egg yolks, leafy green veggies, dried fruits, shellfish, beans, lentils, and artichokes. Pairing iron-rich foods with vitamin C-rich foods will help your body absorb the iron better.[27]

Iron deficiency can affect anyone but it is extremely common among women of childbearing age. Your chiropractor can help you adjust your diet or recommend an iron supplement when necessary.

Vitamin D helps our bodies in the absorption of calcium. Vitamin D also increases bone density and helps prevent bone fractures. Plus, calcium helps regulate the immune system and protects against some types of cancer.

Humans can synthesize their own vitamin D – all it takes is a little sunshine. If you spend a little time in the sun each day, it is unlikely you will be deficient in vitamin D.

People in warm climates rarely have vitamin D problems – it's our neighbors to the north who tend to hibernate through cold, cloudy winters who suffer. If you live far north of the equator, all it really takes is exposing your skin to the sun for about 20 minutes per day (or a little bit longer for older or dark-skinned people) prior to applying sunscreen on most summer days. If you do this, your body will probably synthesize enough vitamin D to last the whole year.[28]

Folic acid is a B vitamin. It helps your body make new cells, repair DNA, and prevent Alzheimer's, anemia, and some forms of cancer.

It is extremely important for pregnant women to get enough folic acid not only while pregnant but prior to pregnancy too. One of the first stages of pregnancy includes the development of the brain and spinal cord, so getting enough folic acid during this process is vital to proper fetal development. Insufficient folic acid has been linked to birth defects including spina bifida and anencephaly.

Veggies and citrus fruits are the best sources of folic acid. Eat plenty of dark leafy greens, asparagus, broccoli, beans, citrus fruits, peas, lentils, avocado, seeds and nuts, carrots, and squash.

Eating a healthy, well-balanced diet can provide you with a strong, energetic, efficient, healthy body. The best way to know if you are getting all the elements that make up a fully functioning healthy body is to discuss your diet with your chiropractor or health care professional. Together, you can ensure that you are providing the optimum fuel to your body.

Your body is designed to heal itself. The nervous system is what controls your immune system. If you're run down, your body is less able to cope with germs and infections. This is when we tend to experience illness or pain. If your nervous system is strong and healthy, your body can deal with injuries and germs better. Chiropractic care focuses on helping you maintain a strong and healthy nervous system, resulting in a healthy body and lifestyle.

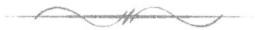

Getting Back to the Basics of Wellness

For a moment, think back to when you were a kid. Chances are that back in elementary school, you had boundless energy. The days were long but it didn't matter - you could probably run around the neighborhood with your friends with hardly a thought of food, pain, or fatigue.

Now maybe you have kids or grandkids, and you watch them go at playtime for hours without a pause – and it's exhausting! We joke about bottling all that energy. We get nostalgic about feeling limitless and free but not enough of us know that there really is a way to regain some of those powerful feelings again.

Wellness is very personal and means different things to different people in terms of preferences and outcomes.

- If you have debilitating back pain, you might feel powerful again if you could get through the day without taking prescription painkillers and suffering through their side effects.
- If your arthritis restricts your daily physical activities, you might feel powerful again if you could go for a

hike again, or knit another afghan without it resulting in days of excruciating joint pain.

- If you suffer from peripheral neuropathy, you might feel powerful again if you could regain sensation in your fingertips again and take up the activities and hobbies you left behind years ago.

Getting older isn't for sissies – but remember that we are lucky to have made it this far!

So what will it take for you to feel energetic and powerful again? There is no correct blanket answer to that question. Every person presents their own set of symptoms, conditions, and preferences. Plus, each person has their own set of goals that will make them feel healthy and happy. All of that makes it complicated to prescribe a roadmap to wellness.

As we discussed in prior chapters, we offer several healing modalities in our office that patients with chronic pain find to be beneficial. Vibration, low-light laser therapy, and electro therapy are a few important resources that many of our patients use every day. We also counsel our patients about the importance of eating a well-balanced diet.

Good nutrition should be considered the cornerstone of any wellness plan. The food you use to fuel your body will make a huge difference when your cells need to repair and regenerate themselves. We promote a diet that's big on unprocessed foods, fruits, vegetables, whole grains, and lean protein. Eating like this gives your body the vitamins, minerals, and antioxidants it needs to stay strong and healthy.

What Else Can I Do to Feel Well?

At the heart of our practice is a busy wellness clinic that offers chiropractic. We strongly believe in the power of a strong, aligned spine that supports a healthy central nervous system. Keeping the spine aligned is achieved through gentle, routine chiropractic adjustments. For most of our patients, one adjustment a week works great. But patients recovering from an accident, illness, infection, or injury sometimes require more frequent adjustments for a period of time.

Regular chiropractic adjustments can not only improve the health of your spine and nervous system but they can also:

- Improve mood
- Improve sleep
- Increase energy
- Decrease pain
- Boost flexibility and mobility
- Stop recurring headaches

One of the most important things chiropractic adjustments do is boost the immune system. This is accomplished by clearing the neural pathways so that the central nervous system can communicate effectively with the immune system (and every other system in your body). This communication is hindered when the spine experiences subluxations, which are misalignments along the spinal column. When the nervous system's pathways are cleared, the effects can be quite powerful:

- Decrease in colds, flu, and other contagious illnesses
- Slash the symptoms of asthma and allergies
- Result in fewer hospital admissions

Unfortunately, most people only think to go to the chiropractor if their back hurts. But we can do so much more together than just fix back pain!

What Does Chiropractic Do for Peripheral Neuropathy?

As you may recall, the treatment modalities we already discussed for peripheral neuropathy were all about rebuilding nerves, growing blood vessels, and improving muscle function. Well chiropractic is all about clearing the way for the nervous system to do its job right. So when your brain can tell those tiny nerve endings that it's time to regrow, all those other efforts we talked about are far more likely to be successful.

In addition to fostering the regrowth of damaged nerves, chiropractic can also unpinch nerves. A pinched nerve can cause numbness and pain, just like peripheral neuropathy. Getting the bones back into their proper places takes pressure off nerves, alleviates pain, and promotes a healthy, active lifestyle. It also gets the joint in the hands, feet or both moving better if affected by neuropathy.

What Should I Do if I Suspect That I Have Peripheral Neuropathy?

The National Institutes of Neurological Disorders and Stroke says that peripheral neuropathy affects roughly 24 million Americans.[29] It's a very common condition among people in certain populations, such as diabetics, cancer patients, and those taking statin medications to lower their cholesterol. Therefore, it's important to know that if you do have peripheral neuropathy, you are certainly not alone.

While the early stages of the symptoms may seem to be just minor irritations, early diagnosis of peripheral neuropathy can prevent the condition from becoming worse. Talk to your doctor right away to diagnose and determine the cause of your peripheral neuropathy. There could be ways to change your medical treatment plan that can reduce your symptoms.

We also strongly recommend visiting our clinic as soon as you can. We offer a variety of treatments that can reduce or even eliminate the pain, numbness, and tingling associated with PN. There is no reason to wait until the problem becomes worse – as soon as you suspect that something is wrong, seek professional help. It's the best way to ensure your health and wellness for many years to come.

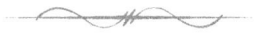

Blueprint to Weight Loss

Blueprint to Weight Loss is a simple, fast, fun weight loss program that allows the patient and the doctor to have an auto-pilot program with fast, permanent results.

It's an easy-to-follow weight loss, detoxification, and healthy living program that is really effective. In fact, we see people lose between half a pound and a pound of fat per day.

Most weight loss programs out there are great but if you follow up with the participants just three months later, the weight is starting to come back, and the results aren't permanent.

This typically happens because most weight loss programs don't address the root causes of weight gain and aren't physician supervised or customized to the specific needs of the client. So, if you want simple, fast, and permanent weight loss, you have to address the root cause of the weight gain. That's why our program doesn't include pills to swallow or any supplements that you have to continue using after you reach your goal.

We have asked hundreds of patients about the root cause of their weight gain and realized that they have no idea. Most of the time we hear things like, "I'm eating too much and moving too little." We wish it was that simple!

The truth is, the root causes of weight gain include:

- candida
- thyroid dysfunction
- metabolism
- hormones
- hypothalamus dysfunction
- stress
- toxicity
- poor food management

1. Candida

The first root cause is candida. Candida is a yeast found in the body, specifically in the gut lining. A little may be relatively harmless but when there is an overgrowth, it starts to cause some serious health issues.

Candida feeds off of sugar and thrives in cool environments in the body. Because of this, it makes you crave sugar and your thyroid begins to come under fire. We will go over this in more detail in a minute.

As candida starts to die off, it releases up to 80 different types of toxins in the body. In order for these toxins to get out of the body, they have to be filtered through the liver.

If the liver is already full of toxins (because of the food we eat,) those extra toxins get stored in the fat cells. Usually, these fat cells start to accumulate around the midsection because of the hormone cortisol that drives them there. Because fat is for protection, the cells will start to harden and not want to release their contents to keep the toxins out of the bloodstream.

That's what's going on when you have stubborn fat. That's the main reason why those fat cells do not want to release their toxins. The kind of fat we're talking about is the kind that won't budge no matter how much you try to work out or work it off. So in order to start getting rid of fat in that area, we have to address the root cause.

The first thing that needs to be done is get the candida under control. Remember, candida is a fungus and yeast that thrives in cool environments. Our bodies are smart enough to use the thyroid to try and turn up our body's temperature to thwart the candida. But, just like anything, if you work overtime, you will eventually burn out.

This will start overworking the thyroid and the thyroid will become sluggish and burn out due to long periods of overworking. This is where a state of hypothyroidism starts to come in, which makes your body a breeding ground for weight gain.

So, we have a specific liquid herbal supplement which kills candida on contact. Once you get that in your system, your sugar cravings will be less intense and less frequent, and you will begin to feel like yourself again (candida can even cause brain fog!)

2. Thyroid dysfunction

So, the second root cause of weight gain is the thyroid. Your thyroid has a big job. The hormones it secretes help maintain a healthy heart rate, maintain healthy skin, and play a crucial role in your metabolism.

When the gland is sluggish, as we just discussed due to candida, it can rob you of your energy, dry out your skin, and make your joints ache. Those are all undesirable symptoms but specifically what we're talking about here is that it can cause dramatic weight gain. That's a lot of grief for such a small gland, isn't it? So, how can we help get the thyroid back to its normal level? We have a unique blend of whole food minerals from sea vegetables that provide natural iodine, and macro- and trace minerals. All of these ingredients work together synergistically to give your thyroid exactly what it needs to release those specific hormones that enable you to have a high metabolic rate. Maintaining a high metabolic rate helps keep your body temperature high enough so that it can start to kill off the terrible candida.

Test your thyroid at home for free.

Before you go to bed, leave a digital thermometer on your bed-side table. First thing in the morning, before even getting out of bed, check your temperature under each arm with the thermometer. If it is below 97.8 degrees, it is a sign of a sluggish thyroid. Do this test three days in a row to get an average.

3. Hormones

Another cause of weight gain is hormones. Hormones give us feedback on things like the feeling of fullness. The key sensations when it comes to hormones are hunger, energy, and cravings. These three things give us clues as to how our hormones are behaving. You cannot lose weight permanently or stay on a good food management plan if your "HEC" (hunger, energy, and cravings) are out of balance.

To combat low hormone levels, we have a topical support. We use a homeopathic liposomal cream. The ingredients in this cream are encapsulated in a specific type of vessel called liposomes. This helps facilitate absorption of the supplement by the body and allows for more of it to be absorbed into the bloodstream and delivered into the cells.

There are four different hormones that affect your weight:

a. **Adiponectin:** Adiponectin is the hormone that tells your body to burn fat for fuel. Multiple studies have shown that the more of this super hormone you have circulating in your bloodstream, the more fat you burn. Research shows that low levels of adiponectin are associated with a higher incidence of obesity.

b. **Cortisol:** Your body produces cortisol in response to stress and ramps you up so you can be ready to fight or flee. With the constant stress in today's hectic world, our cortisol levels are elevated far beyond what we were originally designed to handle. The result, increased sugar cravings, slower metabolism, higher percent of fat stored in midsection, and depression.

c. **Ghrelin:** Ghrelin is called the "Hunger Hormone." The more ghrelin you have in your system, the hungrier you are. If you find yourself fighting cravings and can't seem to stay away from the fridge after dinner, it's probably elevated ghrelin levels. Ghrelin works directly on the hunger center of your brain by activating the brain's reward response to highly addictive sweet, fatty foods.

d. **Insulin:** If you're overweight, there's a good chance that you're experiencing some level of insulin imbalance, resulting in excess glucose, or sugar, in your system. While this doesn't necessarily mean that you're diabetic, it does mean that your body's insulin becomes less effective at lowering your blood sugars. The end result is that most of the carbohydrates you consume get stored as fat.

4. Metabolism

Metabolism is the process by which your body converts what you eat and drink into energy. During this complex biochemical process, calories in food and beverages are combined with oxygen to release energy that your body needs to function.

Even when you are at rest, your body needs energy for all of its hidden functions such as breathing, heartbeat, circulating blood, producing hormones, and growing and repairing cells. The number of calories that your body uses to carry out these functions is called your basal metabolic rate. This is what you might call your "metabolism."

The supplement that we use to help boost metabolism is a specific combination of natural caffeine, flower essence, and white isotopes. It helps raise your metabolic rate without causing jitters or problems sleeping.

Imagine trying to take a tire off of a car. The first turn of the lug nut can be challenging. But once you get it loosened, it becomes much easier. This is what the product does for your metabolism and the reason you don't have to stay on it forever.

Foods that naturally boost your metabolism include:

- almonds
- blueberries
- spinach
- salmon
- turkey

5. Hypothalamus dysfunction

Almost everything that goes on in the body has to do with the hypothalamus, including weight management and controlled weight loss. The hypothalamus is normally not addressed in any weight loss program. Nor are any of the other root causes we have mentioned so far.

Most simply put, when the hypothalamus is broken, food becomes increasingly important because we never end up feeling satisfied with the foods that we have eaten, and we end up eating more and more to try to compensate! From a metabolic standpoint, the hypothalamus not only governs your motivation to eat, it also stimulates hunger and appetite. But most importantly, it controls how satisfying eating is and how deeply the feeling of satiety occurs. This should give us an idea of how important healthy hypothalamus function really is.

We hear so many people say that they never feel satisfied when they are on a weight loss program but that's their hypothalamus talking. We have a way to help you with that in our program. In order to ensure a healthy hypothalamus function, diet is key.

We have a simple food management plan that is specifically designed to provide the correct amount of meats (if you eat them,) vegetables, fruits, and controlling your carb cravings. We also have tools to help you, including measuring spoons and a scale, so you don't have to worry about counting points or calories.

Four things to maintain health hypothalamus health

- exercise regularly
- get enough sleep
- eat healthy fats
- reduce stress

Once you get your hypothalamus functioning properly, it is very important to incorporate these good habits to keep it healthy.

6. Stress

And the last root cause of weight gain is general stress.

When they're on a weight loss program a lot of people get stressed - and we know that stress creates weight gain because of cortisol! So you don't want overall stress when you are trying to lose weight. You will be spinning your wheels if you are on a weight loss program that stresses you out.

Imagine if we could control the stress response by simply reframing our thought process! This is the game-changer with our program. Having the right doctor behind you, the right program in front of you, and 24/7 support around you and that will definitely help neutralize the stress that comes with most other weight loss programs.

Best essential oils to help reduce stress

- lavender
- frankincense
- chamomile

When it comes down to it, we have to get down to the basics and address the root causes that we just discussed to achieve the permanent weight loss that you want. If you love to cook, we have a recipe book with over 100 healthy recipes that can be made in less than ten minutes.

That's the blueprint to weight loss

So, to sum up, we are:

- teaching your mind and body how to burn fat instead of sugar
- supporting you through your journey of finally addressing the root cause of weight gain
- giving you a lifetime program to be sure that the weight stays off
- all while making the program simple, easy, and fun with 24/7 support

Contour Light Therapy

Contour Light is a light emitting diode (LED) system specifically designed to contour the body by losing inches in circumference off specific body areas (waist, hips, thighs, arms, neck) without any pain, downtime, needles or surgery.

Contour Light is composed of four extra large pads that are placed directly to the fatty areas that are resistant to diet and exercise.

How quickly does Contour Light work and what results can I expect?

Results can be seen immediately. Individuals have lost anywhere from two inches to eighteen inches over the course of a series of treatments, though individual results may vary.

How long is a Contour Light treatment and what does it feel like?

You will feel a gentle, warm sensation. You can read, watch television, or take a nap during the 30-minute treatment.

How can you optimize your Contour Light results?

Hydration and exercise are critical. Drink plenty of water (ideally at least eight glasses of eight ounces of water) spread out throughout the day to flush the fat from the system. Diuretics (coffee, alcohol, etc.) are discouraged. You should be active and burn 350 calories every day during their choice of cardio exercise.

What areas of the body can you treat?

Essentially all parts of the body where subcutaneous deposits of fat can be found may be treated with Contour Light, especially those resistant to diet and exercise.

How is Contour Light different from liposuction?

Liposuction is an invasive procedure involving the mechanical removal of fat cells.

By contrast, Contour Light is completely non-invasive and only affects fat cells temporarily. Contour Light does not compete with liposuction; it is simply a body shaping option if you do not wish to undergo a surgical procedure.

Does Contour Light help with loose skin?

Anecdotal evidence suggests that clients undergoing Contour Light have noticed an improvement in skin tone and texture.

Does Contour Light improve the appearance of cellulite?

Anecdotal evidence suggests that clients undergoing Contour Light have noticed an improvement in the appearance of cellulite.

What are the side effects?

There are zero side effects. The treatment is painless and normal activities can be resumed immediately.

How long will results last?

Contour Light does not destroy fat cells but empties them of their contents, which means that fat cells are capable of restoring fat should the client have a chronic caloric imbalance. A balanced diet is the only way to ensure long-term improvement. Clients who eat more calories than they burn will see their improvement decrease over time.

How many treatments will you need?

Normal weight requires 10 to 12 treatments. Overweight requires more than 12 treatments.

Would more treatments lead to better results?

Yes, additional treatments will lead to improved results. An additional series of Contour Light treatments can begin immediately after the first series.

Why should you avoid alcohol during the Contour Light process?

There are three main reasons why alcohol should be avoided with Contour Light:

1. Alcohol is a diuretic and it is critical that the body stays optimally hydrated throughout the treatment program.
2. Alcohol also contains a lot of calories: a five-ounce glass of red wine packs 100 calories! This directly conflicts with the recommendations of the program, which calls for a balanced diet and a healthy lifestyle.
3. Third and most importantly, alcohol is processed as fat by the liver which directly restricts the body's ability to process the newly liberated fat. Once liberated by Contour Light, the fat that is not used up as energy to fuel the body's normal metabolic needs is processed by the liver using enzymes. The total amount of fat being processed at any given time is limited by the amount of enzymes produced by the liver. Alcohol is processed as fat by the liver using the same enzymes.

So, when the liver is busy processing alcohol, it is not able to process the fat liberated by Contour Light. Hence more time/treatments are required to achieve results.

Pre-treatment instructions for best results

1. Eat lightly and drink water: A minimum of 64 ounces of water per day will flush the fat from your system. Divide your body weight by two and this is the number of ounces you should be drinking. Stay hydrated before your treatment and after. Contour Light is attracted to well-hydrated cells.

2. Food limitations: Eat only a light meal or nothing 2 hours before or after your scheduled appointment.
3. Wear comfortable clothing.
4. Do cardio following treatment: Burn 350 calories following your treatment with walking, jogging, stair master, etc. This will burn the fat exactly where you want to. Contour Light is the best personal trainer you can hire. We generally recommend use of a full body vibration plate followed by an energetic cardio workout. The average fat loss is between 40 and 60 grams, which translates into 300 to 500 calories that need to be worked off to maximize your results. The exercise does not have to follow immediately but could be done later on the same day.
5. Follow a low-fat and low-carb diet
6. Avoid alcohol: Alcohol turns into fat and will work against this treatment and will lessen your results. For best results refrain from alcohol on the previous day.
7. Decrease caffeine: Caffeine will dehydrate you which will decrease your results. Only drink the caffeine you need in the morning to avoid "caffeine headache." If possible, completely eliminate caffeine.
8. The small print: Our recommended plan is an initial treatment plan of at least 9-15 visits to get optimum results. If your response to the treatment is favorable, you will have an opportunity to purchase more visits at a discounted rate.

Your first visit will be approximately 30 minutes and will consist of a consultation and an evaluation. We will strive to accommodate your scheduling needs to the best of our ability. Don't forget to ask us about our referral process.

Rules To Optimize Treatment Results

- Keep your regular appointments. Make up your appointment if you miss it. Red light is cumulative and the most significant results appear during the last 25% of treatment.
- Drink plenty of water. 8-10 glasses a day.
- Reduce caloric intake by 500 to 800 calories a day.
- Eat only a light meal or nothing two hours before and two hours after treatment.
- Avoid alcohol during the course of your treatment.
- Do 12 minutes of interval exercise after the light session.
- Do 10 minutes on the whole body vibration plate after the light session.
- Use a liver detox supplement during the course of your treatments.

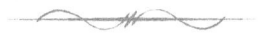

Regenerative Medicine

Regenerative medicine is an interdisciplinary modality that seeks to repair or replace damaged or diseased human cells or tissues to restore normal function. It holds the promise of revolutionizing patient care in the 21st century.

Regenerative medicine may involve the transplantation of stem cells, progenitor cells or tissue, stimulation of the body's own repair processes, or the use of cells as delivery-vehicles for therapeutic agents such as genes and cytokines.

Stem cell research plays a central role in regenerative medicine, which also includes tissue engineering, developmental cell biology, cellular therapeutics, gene therapy, biomaterials, chemical biology and nanotechnology.[30]

Stem cell therapy

It is one of the most advanced options available today to assist you in recovering your health.

Future applications of stem cell therapy include:

- Neurodegeneration such as Alzheimer's disease, Amyotrophic lateral sclerosis, and Parkinson's.[31]

- Brain and spinal cord injury[32]
- Severe heart disease[33]
- Blindness and vision impairment[34]
- Diabetes[35]

In addition, the FDA has approved five hematopoietic stem-cell products derived from umbilical cord blood, for the treatment of blood and immunological diseases.[36]

These undifferentiated stem cells can differentiate to become any type of cell depending on the site of injection. These cells regenerate the tissue, allowing your body to mend from partial tears and other conditions affecting the knees, shoulders, hips, ankles and hands such as partial tears, tendonitis, shoulder pain, knee pain, plantar fasciitis, lateral epicondylitis (tennis elbow) and medial epicondylitis (golfer's elbow).

Stem cell therapy can help you avoid surgery. It is an in-office procedure that takes less than 15 minutes to complete. Stem cell therapy does not need anesthesia and down time. There is practically no recovery time and no adverse effects. Results of significant regeneration are typically seen within 30 days.

Platelet-rich plasma therapy

Platelet-rich plasma (PRP) is a concentrate of platelet-rich plasma protein derived from whole blood, centrifuged to remove red blood cells. It has a greater concentration of growth factors than whole blood, and has been used to encourage a rapid healing response across several specialties, especially dentistry, orthopedics and dermatology.[37]

Platelet-rich plasma therapy (PRP) is a simple yet impactful modality to speed up your recovery. A portion of your own blood is used to isolate platelets, which are then re-injected into the injured area, stimulating healing of ligaments, tendons, muscles and joints.

Prolotherapy

Prolotherapy (proliferation therapy) is an injection-based treatment used in chronic musculoskeletal conditions.[38] Prolotherapy involves the injection of an irritant solution into a joint space,[39] ligament, or tendon to relieve pain.[40] The injection is administered at joints or at tendons where they connect to bone.

The most common solution used is hyperosmolar dextrose. Other commonly used solutions are glycerin, lidocaine (a local anesthetic), phenol, and sodium morrhuate (derived from cod liver oil).

Prolotherapy treatment sessions are generally given in a series ranging from 3 to 6 or more treatments every two to six weeks for several months.[41] However, prolotherapy may be given at less frequent intervals.[42]

Side effects of prolotherapy are mild such as mild pain and irritation at the injection site (often within 72 hours of the injection), numbness at the injection site, or mild bleeding.[43]

Prolotherapy is effective in the treatment of conditions like Achilles tendinopathy, lateral epicondylitis, and knee osteoarthritis.[44, 45]

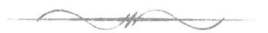

Whole Body Cryotherapy

Cryotherapy is "super-cooling" of the body for therapeutic purposes. Whole-body cryotherapy involves exposing your body to vapors that reach ultra-low temperatures ranging from minus 200 to minus 300 degrees Fahrenheit. You are enclosed in an individual-size enclosure that is open at the top, typically for about three minutes. Your torso and legs are enclosed in the device while the head remains above the enclosure at room temperature.

Since the 1970s when cryotherapy was introduced to treat rheumatoid arthritis, its applications have skyrocketed. A quick, three-minute whole-body cryotherapy session causes a physiological response in the body that penetrates to your core. The blood moves from the extremities inward in an attempt to generate heat, where it is reoxygenated and sent back to the extremities to boost the healing process. It has numerous benefits including:

- pain management of chronic conditions
- athletic performance and recovery
- beauty and anti-aging
- health and wellness

- weight loss
- systemic anti-inflammatory response
- injury recovery and prevention

After the treatment, you will feel increased energy and focus, and improved mood. Whether you are an athlete in search of a superior recovery method, or wanting to get rid of chronic aches and pains, cryotherapy can help. Whole-body cryotherapy can help with the following conditions:

- osteoarthritis
- rheumatoid arthritis
- multiple sclerosis
- ankylosing spondylitis
- chronic pain
- depression and mood disorders
- tendinitis
- bursitis
- fibromyalgia
- joint pain
- muscle soreness
- wrinkles and fine lines
- psoriatic arthritis

When performed in the appropriate and controlled conditions, whole-body cryotherapy is a very safe procedure. Contraindications include cryoglobulinemia, cold intolerance, Raynaud's disease, hypothyroidism, acute respiratory system disorders, heart diseases (unstable angina pectoris, cardiac failure in III and IV stage according to NYHA), purulent-gangrenous skin lesions, sympathetic nervous system neuropathies, local blood flow disorders, cachexia, and hypothermia.[46]

Some applications of whole-body cryotherapy

Whole-body cryotherapy reduces inflammatory responses after heavy physical exercise resulting in decreased sports-induced cell and tissue damage.[47]

Overall, research results indicate that whole-body cryotherapy is effective in reducing the inflammatory process. These results may be explained by vasoconstriction at muscular level, and decrease in pro-inflammatory cytokine activity, and increase in anti-inflammatory cytokines.[48]

For example, three whole-body cryotherapy sessions performed within 48 hours after a strenuous running exercise accelerated recovery from exercise-induced muscle damage to a greater extent than far infrared or passive modalities.[49]

In professional tennis players, whole-body cryotherapy along with moderate-intensity training was more effective for the recovery process than the training alone in the postseason tennis training program.[50]

Autoimmune diseases: 120 patients suffering from primary fibromyalgia (40.7%), rheumatoid arthritis (17.3%), chronic low back pain (16.4%), ankylosing spondylitis (10.9%), osteoarthritis (9.1%), secondary fibromyalgia (3.6%) and other autoimmune diseases reported significant reduction in pain after whole-body cold therapy.[51]

Depression and anxiety: Whole-body cryotherapy is useful as a short-term additional treatment of depression and anxiety. It improved 12 of the 16 items in the Hamilton Depression Rating Scale and 11 of 14 items in the Hamilton Anxiety Rating

Scale. It also improved 6 of the11 items in the life satisfaction scale including physical and mental health, everyday activity, vocational activity, hobbies and general life.[52]

Comparison of whole-body cryotherapy and ice bath

	Whole Body Cryotherapy	Ice Bath
Treatment Delivery	Extreme cold air (-220°F to -280°F)	Cold water(45°F to 60°F)
Resulting Skin Temp	32°F to 35°F	45°F to 60°F
Treatment Time	2 to 3 minutes	15 to 20 minutes
Level of Comfort	High	Low
Response from Body	Vasolidation; Internal Blood Cycle	Warmed blood to peripherals
Enriches Blood	YES	NO
Increases Hemoglobin	YES	NO
Blood Temperature Change	Increased	Decreased
Improves Blood Circulation	YES	NO
Improves Immune System	YES	NO
Risk of Hyperthermia	NO	YES
Release of Endorphins	YES	NO
Time to Return to Exercise	Immediately	12 to 24 hours
Improves Skin Health	YES	NO
Increases Collagen Production	YES	NO

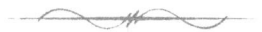

Spinal Vitality and Wellness

If the nerves that exit the lower back and go down to the legs and feet or the nerves that leave the neck and go down into the arms and hands are being compressed, pain, tingling, numbness or other symptoms ensue. Compression in the spine involving the disc and the nerves themselves can cause pain at the spine but not always. The sources of pain can be directly from the disc, or the disc putting pressure on the nerves themselves. Here are the most common ways nerves in the spine can become compressed:

- disc degeneration
- disc bulging
- disc herniation
- osteoarthritis
- inflammation
- infection
- misalignment of the spine
- tumors of the spine
- scoliosis or curvatures
- rheumatoid arthritis

Surgeons perform surgical spinal decompression and remove the bone or disc around the spinal cord or the nerves that exit the spine. In our clinic, we use a non-invasive technique called non-surgical spinal decompression therapy.

Benefits of spinal decompression therapy:

- reduces disc pressure
- enhances disc healing
- inhibits leakage of disc material
- pulls disc material that has protruded back into the disc (vacuum effect)
- pumps in oxygen, and other nutrients into the discs and pumps out waste products like carbon dioxide

Most common indications for spinal decompression therapy:

- sciatica
- herniated disc
- degenerative disc disease
- facet joint syndrome (osteoarthritis)
- peripheral neuropathy from compressed nerves

Relative contraindications for spinal decompression therapy include:

- osteoporosis
- severe arthritis
- spondylolisthesis
- paralysis
- disc fragmentation
- disc calcification
- surgical spinal appliances

If you have one or more of the above relative contraindications, it doesn't mean you can't have the therapy, it only means we need to be cautious and start the therapy gradually and gently.

Procedure:

You lie either on your back or belly. A strap is wrapped around the pelvis and connected to the cable of the spinal decompression machine. Another strap is used to hold the upper body in place while the lower body is being pulled. A computer is programmed considering a patient's height, weight, age, body type and other factors such as diabetes and osteoporosis.

The machine always starts out with a very light force, usually 5 pounds, and pulls for around 30 seconds. It then takes most of the weight off, allowing a resting period for 30 seconds. Next, a larger force, about 10 pounds is applied for 30 seconds, followed by rest. The force is gradually and progressively increased with alternate rest periods until the maximum force is reached. Then, the whole process is reversed, and the force is progressively reduced.

For cervical (neck) spinal decompression therapy, smaller forces are used. The unit's cervical device exerts a gently pull using cranial bolsters.

Spinal Traction

It is continuous pulling of the spine with the same amount of force. It is done using an inversion table. Your ankles are strapped into the table in the upright position and then the table is slowly rotated to the inverted position (upside down).

To start with, this is done for no more than 30 seconds and gradually increased to a few minutes. This therapy can help with muscle spasms and even disc pain.

The main difference between spinal traction and spinal decompression therapy is the application of force. Traction uses a continuous force, usually, your body weight. However, in spinal decompression therapy, the machine machines varies the forces.

Scientific research on spinal decompression therapy

Non-surgical spinal decompression was done on 30 patients with low back pain who underwent a six-week protocol of non-surgical spinal decompression. CT scans before and after treatment showed an increase in the height of the affected discs. They also reported reduction of pain.[53]

Sixty-seven patients with chronic low back pain and radiologic evidence of a herniated disc underwent an eight-week course of non-surgical vertebral axial decompression therapy. Significant improvement was seen in pain rating and activity-limitation at discharge, 30, and 180 days after treatment.[54]

The purpose of this study was to see if patients responded to two different protocols of vertebral axial decompression. Patients who failed standard medical physical therapy underwent two different protocols of vertebral axial decompression. Those who did 18 sessions of non-surgical vertebral axial decompression achieved a higher percent of remission (76%) than those who did only 9 (43%).[55]

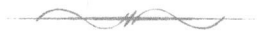

Hyperbaric Oxygen Therapy

Hyperbaric oxygen therapy is inhalation of 100 percent pure oxygen in a pressurized chamber, where air pressure is increased to three times the normal pressure. It is a simple, painless, drug-free, and non-invasive treatment.

During hyperbaric oxygen therapy, oxygen dissolves in all of the body's fluids and reaches all parts of the body, including those where the blood circulation is impaired. The extra oxygen reaches damaged tissues and boosts the body's healing process naturally and with minimal side effects. Hyperbaric oxygen therapy helps to heal damaged capillary walls, prevents plasma leakage and reduces swelling.

Hyperbaric oxygen therapy is used to treat the following conditions:

- severe anemia
- brain abscess
- arterial gas embolism (air bubbles in your blood vessels)
- burns
- decompression sickness
- carbon monoxide poisoning
- crushing injury
- sudden deafness

- gangrene
- infection of skin or bone causing tissue death
- non-healing wounds, such as a diabetic foot ulcer
- radiation injury
- skin graft or skin flap at risk of tissue death
- sudden and painless vision loss

Hyperbaric oxygen therapy is an outpatient procedure and doesn't require hospitalization. The number of sessions depends on your medical condition. Hyperbaric oxygen therapy alone can effectively treat decompression sickness, arterial gas embolism and severe carbon monoxide poisoning. However, for treatment of other conditions, it is used with other therapies and drugs.[56]

Hyperbaric oxygen may be used in the treatment of conditions such as stroke, traumatic brain injury, sports injuries, Lyme disease, migraine, multiple sclerosis and other neurodegenerative disorders.

A study on the effect of hyperbaric oxygen on mild traumatic brain injury reported significant improvement in cognitive function and quality of life as well as elevated brain activity. The study was carried out on 56 patients with mild traumatic brain injury and prolonged post-concussion syndrome, 1 to 5 years after injury. There was significant improvement in cognitive function and quality of life after 40 HBOT sessions of 60 minutes each, with 100% oxygen at 1.5 ATA (atmospheres absolute).[57]

Another study on 74 patients who suffered stroke 6–36 months earlier and had at least one motor dysfunction reported significant improvements such as renewed use of language, enhanced sensation, and reversal of paralysis of all patients.

The results indicate that hyperbaric oxygen therapy can lead to significant neurological improvements in post stroke patients even at chronic late stages.[58]

Oxygen multi-step therapy (exercise with oxygen therapy) combines oxygen therapy, drugs that facilitate intracellular oxygen turnover, and physical exercise adapted to individual performance levels. Breathing pure oxygen while exercising dramatically increases the amount of oxygen absorbed into the blood circulation and tissue fluids.

There are three systems that deliver different levels of oxygen to the body:

1. **Hyperbaric oxygen therapy** delivers about 20 liters of oxygen per minute and requires about 20 to 60 hours of therapy.
2. **Exercise with oxygen therapy** delivers about 5 to 10 liters of oxygen per minute and requires about 36 hours of therapy.
3. **Live Oxygen** delivers more than 50 liters of oxygen per minute and requires 15 minutes or less of therapy.

Hyperbaric oxygen therapy is a very safe procedure. Some people may feel slightly uncomfortable pressure in their ears during the therapy but most people tolerate it well and enjoy their one-hour sessions reading, watching videos, or just relaxing.

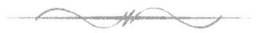

Knee Pain

Knee pain is a common complaint that can affect people of all ages. The location and severity of knee pain may vary, depending on the cause of the problem.

Knee pain can be caused by

1. Knee injuries:

- Injury to the ACL (anterior cruciate ligament), which is a ligament that connects your shinbone to your thighbone. It is common in sports like basketball and soccer that require sudden changes in direction.
- Fractures of the bones of the knee, including the kneecap during falls or road accidents.
- Injury to the meniscus, which is the cartilage between your shinbone and thighbone. It can be torn if you twist your knee while bearing weight on it.
- Inflammation of the knee bursa, which is a small sac of fluid on the outer side of your knee joint.
- Inflammation of patellar tendons, which connects the quadriceps muscle on the front of the thigh to the shinbone, can affect runners, cyclists, and track and field athletes.

2. Arthritis:

- Osteoarthritis, which is the most common type of arthritis, caused by wear-and-tear of tissues in your knee.
- Rheumatoid arthritis is a chronic autoimmune disorder.
- Infective arthritis is usually accompanied by swelling, pain, redness and. fever.
- Pseudogout is caused by calcium-containing crystals in the joint fluid. It affects the knees most commonly.
- Gout is caused by deposition of uric acid crystals in the knee joint.

3. Other causes:

- Loose body in the knee caused by a small broken piece of bone or cartilage in the joint space.
- Iliotibial band syndrome, caused by tightness of the iliotibial band, which extends from the outside of your hip to the outside of your knee.
- Dislocation of the kneecap, usually to the outer side of your knee.
- Foot or hip disorders can affect your knee joints because of altered gait.

Risk factors for knee pain

- Excess weight increases stress on your knee joints because they are weight-bearing joints, especially when climbing stairs. It also increases the risk of osteoarthritis.
- Tight or weak knee muscles and ligaments increase the risk of knee injuries.

- Games like skiing, basketball, and football as well as long distance running increase the risk of knee injury.
- Previous knee injury increases the likelihood of knee injuries and arthritis in the future.[59]

Indications for seeking chiropractic for your knee pain

Knee pain can affect all your activities like walking to your car, climbing the stairs, or even getting out of bed. Is the knee pain severe enough to limit your daily activities? Are the pain medication and other conventional modalities of treatment ineffective? Instead of deciding to reduce your activities, take more painkillers or tolerate the pain, why not try chiropractic treatment?

A chiropractor will not only address the causes of the pain in and around the knee but will also investigate if other disorders in other parts of the body may be the real or contributory cause of the knee pain.

For example, the knee pain may be a compensation for a mechanical disorder in the lower back, a common condition that may not be diagnosed by conventional medical practitioners. If the lower back is mechanically dysfunctional, it can place additional stress on one or both knees. It's important to address the source of the problem instead of merely managing the knee symptoms. Also, limitation of hip movements could place excessive strain on the knees.

The right chiropractic care includes a combination of techniques to alleviate your pain and to address the underlying issues that may be causing the knee pain. There are usually several modalities of therapy like:

- ice application to reduce knee inflammation
- massage therapy to improve the range of motion
- chiropractic manipulation
- mobilization techniques in the area of restricted movement in the knee as well as surrounding joints.

These modalities not only help to reduce knee pain but also increase the range of movement and improve the function of your knees.

Another treatment option is stem cell therapy. Stem cells are undifferentiated cells that can differentiate and turn into any type of cell depending on the site of injection. These cells regenerate the tissue. If injected into the knees, they allow your knees to mend tears and other conditions.

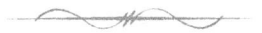

Plantar Fasciitis

Plantar fasciitis is a condition characterized by inflammation of the plantar fascia, a thick band of tissue that runs across the bottom of your foot and connects your heel bone to your toes. It is one of the commonest causes of heel pain.

Symptoms: Plantar fasciitis causes stabbing pain in the bottom of your foot near the heel. The pain is most severe with the first few steps in the morning. However, it can also be triggered by long periods of standing or rising from sitting. The pain is usually worse after exercise, not during it. As you move more, the pain usually decreases. It is more common in runners, overweight people and those who wear shoes with poor support.

Causes: Plantar fasciitis can arise without an obvious cause. Usually, the plantar fascia acts like a shock-absorber and supports the arch in your foot. If there is excessive stress, it can get injured. Repetitive stretching and tearing can cause the fascia to become inflamed.

Risk factors

- Age: Plantar fasciitis is most common between the ages of 40 and 60.

- Exercise: Activities such as long-distance running, jumping activities, and aerobic dance, which place excessive stress on your heel and attached tissues.
- Foot mechanics: flat-feet, a high arch or an abnormal pattern of walking.
- Obesity: Excess body weight put extra stress on your plantar fascia.
- Occupations: Jobs that require you to spend most of your work hours walking or standing on hard surfaces.

Complications: Changing the way you walk to minimize the pain caused by plantar fasciitis may lead to foot, knee, hip or back problems. If you don't seek timely treatment, you may get chronic heel pain, which will make walking painful.

Diagnosis is based on the medical history and physical examination. The location of pain and tenderness in your foot can help to determine its cause. Usually no tests are necessary. However, your doctor might suggest X-rays or MRI to rule out other problems, such as stress fractures, heel spurs or pinched nerves.

Modalities of treatment

Most people who have plantar fasciitis recover with conservative treatments, including rest, ice application to the painful area and stretching. However, full recovery may take a few months. If the pain is very severe, you may have to take painkillers like ibuprofen to reduce the pain and inflammation.

Stretching and strengthening exercises or use of specialized devices may provide symptom relief. These include:

- Physical therapy includes a series of exercises to stretch the plantar fascia and Achilles tendon. Strengthening your lower leg muscles helps to stabilize your ankles and feet. You may also need to apply athletic tape to support the bottom of your foot.

- Night splints that stretch your calf and the arch of your foot while you sleep. This holds the plantar fascia and Achilles tendon in a lengthened position overnight and facilitates stretching.
- Orthotics are arch supports that help to distribute pressure to your feet more evenly.

Lifestyle and home remedies

- Lose weight if you're overweight or obese to minimize stress on your plantar fascia.
- Choose supportive shoes. Buy shoes with low heels, good arch support and shock absorbency. Avoid high heels. Don't walk barefoot, especially on hard surfaces.
- Don't wear worn-out athletic shoes. Replace your old athletic shoes before they stop supporting and cushioning your feet.
- Choose low-impact sports such as swimming or bicycling, instead of walking or jogging.
- Ice application. Hold a cloth-covered ice pack over the area of pain for 15 to 20 minutes three or four times a day or after activity. Or try ice massage. Freeze a water-filled paper cup and roll it over the site of discomfort for about five to seven minutes. Regular ice massage can help reduce pain and inflammation.
- Stretch your arches. Do simple home exercises that stretch your plantar fascia, Achilles tendon, and calf muscles.[60]

Benefits of Chiropractic Care for Plantar Fasciitis

Chiropractic care can address some of the factors that may be causing or worsening plantar fasciitis.

Posture adjustment: Chiropractic care can help you deal with bad posture. Your gait and the impact of your feet while walking can cause or worsen plantar fasciitis. We can help to improve your posture, which will improve the way your feet feel when you stand or walk.

Alignment correction: If your weight isn't balanced across your feet, you may suffer from plantar fasciitis in one foot more than the other. We can help to correct the alignment and balance of your body so that the weight is distributed evenly. This allows the affected foot to heal more quickly and reduces recurrence of the pain.

Pain relief: Chiropractic care can also help to reduce aches and pains in your back, neck, and shoulders. This will help you to feel more positive about your health, and encourage you to do the simple exercises that will reduce the pain of planter fasciitis.

We would like you to take a holistic approach to your health, including plantar fasciitis. If you suffer from bad posture, obesity or an unbalanced alignment, we may be able to help you.

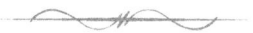

Biohacking

Biohacking or bio optimization is the use of nutrition and technology to improve your ability to heal and your performance in general. Biohacking means finding new and innovative ways to improve your biological health and wellbeing.

All of us need to use biohacking because of the toxic environment that we are exposed to. Pollution, global warming and the unremitting stress of our modern lifestyle is degrading our DNA and adversely affecting our health. Biohacking may help us not just to sustain ourselves but to optimize our lifestyle and health.

A simple biohack is to go outside and stand in sunlight for 20 minutes. This should be done preferably in the morning or evening, when the sunlight is not too strong. Sunlight helps to increase vitamin D synthesis, which is really important for optimal way. This is the best way to prevent Vitamin D deficiency.

Sleep biohack

Lack of sleep affects overall health and may lead to chronic health problems such as mental fatigue, low immunity, obesity, diabetes, and heart disease.

One of the main factors that affect the quality of your sleep is exposure to artificial blue light, especially in the evening. Artificial lighting and electronic devices emit light of a blue wavelength, which tricks our brains into thinking that it is daytime.

Blue light hampers the production of melatonin and disrupts our circadian rhythm. It can also cause photoreceptor damage to your eyes.

One way to decrease blue light in the evening is to use an app called flux (https://justgetflux.com/). This downloadable program automatically adapts the color of your computer's display to the time of day, warm at night and like sunlight during the day. So it not only makes you sleep better but also makes your computer look better. You can buy blue light blocking glasses or screen for TV viewing at night.

By the way, it was thought that the switch to outdoor LED lights would give us less light pollution. However, research led by Christopher Kyba has found that overall light levels went up by 2.2% per year, with some countries using 150% more light. Unfortunately, when lighting is cheaper, we tend to use more light. If we don't make a real effort to control light levels, we are in danger of losing our night.[61]

Some other biohacks that you can do yourself include

- drink filtered water
- walk barefoot on earth or sand
- spend time in nature
- improve your circadian rhythm
- replace all toxic cleaning products in your home with non-toxic ones

- calm the mind with a daily breathing, meditation or prayer practice
- replace all GMO foods with organic, whole food
- minimize processed foods, especially those containing simple sugars and trans fat (anti-inflammatory diet)
- do high-intensity intermittent exercise regularly
- use blood flow restriction training
- practice daily gratitude
- volunteer with an organization that you are passionate about
- improve postural awareness
- follow your passion
- give 3-6 second hugs and really feel a connection with that person
- re-wire negative thought patterns
- maintain healthy relationships with family and friends

Fortunately, we are more willing to take responsibility for our health instead of depending on the conventional medical system, which is not working so well. Seen from this perspective, chiropractic care is itself an effective biohack.

Examples of effective biohacks in chiropractic care include:

- low-level light therapy or photobiomodulation
- LED light therapy (light-emitting diodes)
- hyperbaric oxygen therapy
- red light therapy
- contour light
- whole-body cryotherapy
- fascial stretch therapy
- sequential pulse technology
- massage therapy
- nerve re-education

- stem cell therapy
- platelet-rich plasma therapy
- compression therapy
- cupping therapy
- Kinesio Taping® Method

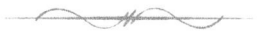

Train the Mind, the Body Will Follow

"There is no other area of American life where we collectively accept such a bad deal. We spend more than any other nation on our military, but our military is unquestionably the mightiest in the world. We spend the most on our universities, but our universities are the best on the planet. But we spend the most on our health care—twice as much as anyone else—and our health system is mediocre-to-poor, with 47 million of us lacking the insurance necessary to easily access it." Ezra Klein[62]

The U.S. does not have a health care system; it has a disease-management system largely dependent on expensive drugs and invasive surgeries. The mission of the U.S. healthcare system seems to be to maximize profits rather than helping people maintain or regain their health. The more you take responsibility for your own health by nurturing your body, the less you will need to rely on this "disease care" system.[63]

Five science-backed ways to take responsibility for your own health

The following five self-care modalities will boost not only your health but also your brain power:

1. **Healthy nutrition:** A nutritious diet is vital for physical and mental health. Minimize sugar and processed foods and eat more fresh vegetables and whole foods.

2. **Regular exercise:** The most effective exercise is high-intensity interval exercise (HIIT). Other recommended exercises include swimming, Pilates, yoga, strength training, and brisk walking. A sedentary lifestyle increases the risk of obesity, heart disease, and premature death. So, in addition to regular exercise, you need to be active throughout the day.

3. **Restful sleep:** Many people worry about the duration of sleep but the quality of that sleep is more important. During quality sleep state (delta state), the body repairs and rebuilds body tissues, including brain tissue. Regular good-quality sleep is crucial for neural functions such as learning, memory, and neuroplasticity. For even greater benefit, take a short mid-day nap. Even 20 minutes is sufficient to refresh the mind and improve productivity.

4. **Mental stimulation:** Commit to learning something new every day and become a lifelong student. Engaging in cognitively demanding activities helps to stretch and expand all function of the brain such as focus, memory, and learning. A 2015 study of people aged 85 and older concluded that those who used a computer late in life and engaged in artistic and social activities had a lower risk of mild cognitive impairment.[64]

5. **Positive attitude:** A positive attitude includes positive mental qualities like cheerfulness, gratitude, empathy, compassion, forgiveness, and goodwill practices such as mindfulness and generosity. A positive outlook helps to improve your general health and quality of life.

In addition to self-care, it is important to seek proper health care from qualified health professionals.

Integrative medicine is a better alternative to the current healthcare system, as it offers a combination of conventional medical therapies and complementary or alternative therapies for which there is high-quality scientific evidence for safety and effectiveness. Integrative medicine is healing-oriented medicine that takes account of the whole person, including all aspects of lifestyle. It emphasizes the therapeutic relationship between practitioner and patient, is informed by evidence, and makes use of all appropriate therapies.[65]

There are many different aspects to being healthy and none can be compromised. With so many options available, we can help you discover true health. Our team includes a chiropractor, nurse practitioner and medical doctor in addition to our highly qualified, knowledgeable support staff.

Though we are not against traditional medicine when it is required, we feel that many of these options may interfere with your natural healing abilities or simply cover up your symptoms temporarily. Ultimately, we want to stimulate your body's healing process without needing to resort to potentially hazardous medications and surgery.

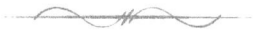

Our Illness to Wellness Seminars

These seminars include management of the following conditions:

- Peripheral Neuropathy
- Weight Loss
- Spinal Vitality
- Knee Pain

PERIPHERAL NEUROPATHY

What is peripheral neuropathy?

As already explained in this book, peripheral neuropathy is a condition where nerves are damaged causing weakness, burning pain, numbness, tingling, and debilitating balance problems.

Poor blood flow to the nerves, toxic levels of sugar in the blood (diabetes), chronic infections, pesticide exposure and genetic variants are a few of the causes of this debilitating condition. The cause is different for every patient and it must be discovered to help the nerves heal.

Another common cause of nerve damage is auto-immunity. Auto-immune diseases are conditions where the immune system mistakenly starts to attack the body. So, the immune system may damage nerves resulting in peripheral neuropathy. This is why thorough testing plays a vital role in the diagnosis and treatment of peripheral neuropathy.

Can peripheral nerves heal?

Yes! It is well established in the scientific literature that peripheral nerves can and do heal. The key is to eliminate the cause of the nerve damage so that nerves can start to heal. Once we discover and treat the underlying cause of the neuropathy and provide proper support to the nerves, it optimizes the ability of the nerves to heal.

In order to effectively heal nerve damage, four factors must be determined:

- What is the underlying cause of the nerve damage?
- How severe is the nerve damage?
- What types of nerve fibers are damaged?
- How much treatment will the nerves require to heal?

Treatment

The treatment that we provide has four main goals...

1. Optimize the environment within the body for nerve healing.
2. Increase blood flow to the nerves.
3. Stimulate the nerves that are damaged to reduce pain and improve balance.
4. Decrease brain-based pain.

Our exclusive treatment system increases blood flow to the nerves in the feet and/or hands, which helps to rejuvenate nerves naturally and has returned many of our patient's feet and/or hands to normal (see testimonials below). No surgery. No addictive medications.

State of the art technology

Our proprietary and comprehensive treatment program utilizes up to eight different modern technologies and is unlike any treatment program you may have already experienced. One of the treatments technologies we use to increase blood flow is our new low-level light Therapy (LLLT).

LLLT is one of the most powerful non-surgical lasers and it gets results. The light therapy signals vascular endothelial growth factor, which stimulates the formation of new blood vessels (angiogenesis). Angiogenesis helps to repair nerve damage. These new blood vessels develop around the peripheral nerves and provide them with the proper nutrients to heal and repair.

We also use state of the art digital electrotherapeutic stimulation to assist in the growth of the nerves called Nerve ReEducation. This is used by the Cancer Treatment Centers of America to repair and rebuild damaged nerves after chemotherapy. Nerve ReEducation can even be done at home, so therapy can be done daily. It provided immediate pain relief and restoration of normal sensation.

Nerve cells need two things to heal: fuel and activation

This makes the combination of high-powered low-level light therapy (fuel) and Nerve ReEducation (activation) the perfect 1-2 punch for nerve regeneration.

The amount of treatment needed to allow the nerves to recover varies from person to person and can only be determined after a detailed neurological and vascular evaluation.

WEIGHT LOSS

Trying to shed stubborn pounds can be an exercise in frustration. With so many different diets available today it can be difficult to know what works and what doesn't. We've found that the majority of our patients want to lose a few pounds and get nutrition counseling to improve their health.

At **CryoNext Integrative Healthcare**, we are pleased to offer patients a specific diet plan tailored to meet their unique needs and goals. The Blueprint to Weight Loss is a simple, fast, fun weight loss program that allows the patient and the doctor to have an auto-pilot program with fast, permanent results. It's an effective and easy-to-follow weight loss, detoxification, and healthy living program. In fact, we see people lose between half a pound and a pound of fat per day.

If you want simple, fast, and permanent weight loss, you have to address the root cause of the weight gain. That's why our program doesn't include pills to swallow or supplements that you have to continue using after you reach your goal.

Whether you are an athlete who wants to decrease your body fat percentage and add muscle mass or someone who wants to lose those extra pounds of fat and keep them off permanently, we offer solutions that work.

SPINAL VITALITY

Each of us is different, and the approach to health care should be unique, too. We use numerous techniques, including both manual and instrument-based methods. Our goal is to tailor each chiropractic treatment to you.

If the nerves that exit the spine at the neck or the lower back are compressed, it can result in pain, tingling, numbness or other symptoms. Surgeons may treat spinal nerve compression with surgical spinal decompression, in which they remove the bone or disc around the spinal cord or the nerves that exit the spine. If you want to avoid the inconvenience, expense, and complications of surgery, you can opt for non-surgical spinal decompression therapy.

Non-surgical spinal decompression therapy reduces disc pressure, enhances disc healing, inhibits leakage of disc material, pulls disc material that has protruded back into the disc (vacuum effect), pumps in oxygen, and other nutrients into the discs and pumps out waste products like carbon dioxide.

This therapy is useful in conditions like sciatica, herniated disc, degenerative disc disease, facet joint syndrome (osteoarthritis), peripheral neuropathy from compressed nerves.

In addition to nerve compression, chiropractic care has been shown to be effective for treating conditions like auto accident injuries, headaches, migraines, neck pain, mid-back pain, low back pain, shoulder pain, hip pain, neuropathy, sprains, strains, sports injury, sciatica, scoliosis, asthma, surgery prevention, blood pressure, neurological conditions, whiplash, frozen shoulder, fibromyalgia, and athletic performance and recovery.

Everything in our body is controlled by the brain, and the brain is able to communicate with each part through the nervous system. Chiropractic care assures that this vital communication system operates optimally, therefore, allowing the body to do what it was designed to and heal itself.

The source of any interference with your nervous system is located and eliminated with highly effective and specific chiropractic adjustments, which restores the brain-body communication and kick-starts the healing process.

Chiropractic care also provides added benefits such as reduced stress, decreased joint aches, greater energy, restful sleep, enhanced mood, and increased focus.

KNEE PAIN

Knee pain is a common complaint that can affect people of all ages. Knee pain can be caused by injuries, inflammation, arthritis, and other disorders. The severity of knee pain may vary, depending on the cause of the problem.

Knee pain can adversely affect all your daily activities and work responsibilities. Therefore, it's vital to address the source of the problem instead of merely managing your knee symptoms. It can be frustrating if rest and painkillers are not able to relieve your knee pain.

Chiropractic care can address the real and contributory causes of the knee pain not only in and around the knee but also in other parts of the body. We use several therapies that quickly relieve your knee pain as well as treat the underlying causes of your knee pain.

That modalities we use include ice application, massage therapy, chiropractic manipulation and mobilization techniques, which increase the range of movement and improve the function of your knees.

Another treatment option is stem cell therapy. Stem cells are undifferentiated cells that can differentiate and turn into any type of cell depending on the site of injection. These cells regenerate the tissue. When injected into the knees, they allow your knees to mend tears and other conditions.

For a limited time, we are offering our Illness to Wellness seminars for FREE. At these seminars, we will discuss your symptoms, medical history, treatment options, and whether this treatment is the right fit for you.

Contact us today to book a seat at one of our free luncheons.

Visit: cryonextintegrative.com/contact-us or call (407) 890-9651.

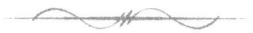

Testimonials

"Great place! Dr. Abraham really does care about his patients. I look forward to coming here at least once a month."

–Ehab K.

"Best chiropractor in town! Dr. Abraham has been great and has gotten me feeling much better following my car accident. Highly recommend!"

–Amany T.

"Beautiful office and incredible technology. Super friendly and knowledgeable staff. Dr. Abraham took a lot of time in the consultation to answer all my questions. I'm very happy to start care and use all the modalities they have. Highly recommend!"

–Heidi F.

"Dr. Abraham and CryoNext have been pretty great. Their staff was very helpful and discerning. I'd recommend to anyone looking for a chiropractor. They also have all the latest and coolest tech in sports recovery. Really glad to have found them."

–Michael R.

"Very warm welcoming staff! I walked in absolutely sore and left feeling better than ever. Definitely will be returning soon."

–Vincent L.

"Dr. Abraham stayed with me for four hours to help solve my back and neck issues. He made sure all of my questions were answered and that I left feeling better than when I came in. I've never had a better chiropractic experience."

–Katie S.

"If you are serious about wellness and recovery, this is where you need to be. One cryo session or compression therapy will take me from excruciating and to pain-free. Add this to your weekly fitness or physical therapy routine, and you will see results."

–Megan Y.

"Amazing experience. So different than any chiropractor I've been to. I feel great! Thank you Dr. Abraham!"

–Joseph A.

"Went to check out cryotherapy for the first time and it was fantastic. All my muscle soreness and joint pain from day to day life went away and it only took 3 minutes. Dr. Abraham and his staff are all very knowledgeable in all treatment methods and have the newest equipment to go with the newest therapy options."

–David R.

"Tried the cryotherapy for the first time today. It worked wonders on my knee. Dr. Abraham is very knowledgeable and has a great passion for his practice."

–Troy B.

"Stopped in for my first Cryotherapy therapy session and was amazed by the results, and the extremely knowledgeable staff. The team here is highly motivated. I had some pain in my knees from my current training regimen, but the Cryotherapy not only removed knee ailments, it also refreshed my entire body. Looking forward to coming back!"

–Matthew G.

Neuropathy Testimonials

"After 31 visits, I was 90-95% cured & I am very fortunate that I came to Blueprint to Healthcare."

–Bill M.

"After only 2 treatments I was able to sleep at night without socks which had been one of my big problems because my feet had been so cold."

–Mickey W.

"I was taking pain medication every day, after 12 visits I stopped taking pain medication. I had no symptoms at night and I did not need sleeping aids anymore. I am extremely happy with my choice to begin the program."

–Rosanna V.

"I have gone from 44% sensory loss down to 15% sensory loss halfway through the program. I'm getting better and I feel a whole lot better."

–Kim M.

"I saw an ad for neuropathy which intrigued me because I was developing neuropathy in my feet and legs. I saw my podiatrist and he confirmed that I have neuropathy. So, I decided to try the program; I had always had trouble with my legs particularly. I could not sleep at night because my legs bothered me so much – in less than 2 weeks I was beginning to sleep through the night!"

–Bob B.

"I came here because of the numbness in my feet, it was all over the top and bottom of my feet as well as my toes. I've been on the program awhile now and all I have is a little bit of numbness so it is definitely working. I would encourage anyone to come here and visit with them. I have been very happy and I believe their maintenance program will help me as well!"

–Matt B.

"Over 5 years ago, I was told by a well-respected neurologist that "nothing can be done other than take B12 and be careful not to fall". I heard about this program at a local rotary meeting, thought I would give it a try...fully expecting a similar situation because of my age. To my surprise after testing, I knew there was potential that I could really get some help. I am now in my 8th week of therapy and the results have been amazing. No longer have tingling sensation or pain."

–Burnell S.

"I have been coming to Blueprint to Healthcare for about a week and half now. Since then I have lost nine pounds sticking to the nutrition plan. I have such bad feet problems, back pain, neck pain, and hand pain that's why I decided to come...since I've been coming, I have already seen quite a bit of difference in this short amount of time. I can't believe the progress I've had in such a short amount of time."

–Ann R.

"My feet have been dead for quite some time. Two different times in my pick-up, I couldn't feel my accelerator. We started the treatment and about 3-4 weeks into the program, after beginning the home treatment...I could feel the carpet when I was walking and that was the first time I had done that in quite some time."

–Mark O.

"I was having pretty bad neuropathy and it was continuing to get worse after seeing medical doctors, they were just giving me some pain pills and vitamin B12 shots. I decided I needed to do something better & be proactive. This will be my third week and between all the treatments they do here, I am already improving – I'm down to one incident a week and I was having 5-6 incidents a day."

–Kelly C.

"Neuropathy was effecting my life pretty bad for almost a year now, to the point where I was in pain most of the time. Since I've been coming here for 3 or 4 sessions now, I have already noticed a lot of difference and I am already feeling a lot better.

–Jesse R.

"I came here very apprehensive. I have been coming only a few weeks now and I have already regained so much strength in my left leg which was the problem. I barely use my cane at all now – just for a little security. I just can't believe how well I am doing after only being treated for a short amount of time!"

–Dorothy C.

"I have suffered from neuropathy for at least three years, I have been completing treatment here and it has already been successful. I can sleep at night without my feet burning and hurting!"

–Betty P.

"I came to Blueprint to Neuropathy because I have neuropathy and it is effecting my golf game. I have been coming about five weeks and I can already tell some improvement in the bottom of my feet."

–Gary C.

"I am relatively new to the program, this is only my third visit. I have already gone from a pain level of 8 to a pain level of 2!"

– Kim N.

"I have been coming about 6 weeks. When I came in, I had severe pain all the way from my hip down to my big toe. As of today, I am able to wiggle my big toe and I have feeling in it! I have NO more pain in my hips or legs. Overall, my time spent here has been well worthwhile! I must say that the staff has been very professional, helpful, and encouraging."

–Nell M.

"I am in my 3rd week of my treatment, when I came in, my left foot was killing me and my right foot was not far behind it. I was asked to rate my pain on a level of 1 – 10 during my consultation and I have been at a level 10 for about three or four months now. My pain level now is nearly gone completely."

–James F.

"I came here after seeing the ad in the paper, I decided to come in because of my neuropathy being so bad. It took a little bit of work but everything they have done here for me has been very great. The staff here is very nice which helps a lot when coming in for treatment."

–Everisto M.

CryoNext Reviews

"Very friendly and knowledgeable staff, Dr. Abraham was amazing and helped me get back to 100% after my car accident! The Cryo machine also helped alleviate a lot of pain, I would definitely recommend this office to all my friends!"

–Mina H.

"If you are serious about wellness and recovery, this is where you need to be. One cryo session or compression therapy will take me from excruciating and to pain-free. Add this to your weekly fitness or physical therapy routine, and you will see results."

–Megan Y.

"I have been coming here for over 2 weeks now and I'm learning so much about the different ways to optimize my body's performance to do what it's naturally designed to do... to heal itself. As a patient diagnosed with rheumatoid arthritis 25 years ago, I am finding new ways to manage my pain and care for myself from the inside out. Combined with proper diet, exercise and sleep, I have chosen, (after trying the conventional way of taking heavy duty prescribed meds under the care of a rheumatologist) a better way that truly makes sense to me. With the help of Dr. Abraham and the knowledgeable staff at Cryonext Integrative, I've been able to feel the difference in as little as 15 days. I plan to continue my treatments for as long as I can. I've tried other places, but nothing compares to the vibrant energy, the friendliest staff and the overall awesome service I get from Cryonext Integrative. It's the future of healthcare. I know I'm a fan!"

–Jonalyn P.

"Cryotherapy definitely changed my view on therapy itself. One of the most state of the art facilities that I've been too and very personal, Dr. Abraham is hands on and well educated on all of his equipment. 100% recommend!"

–Jermaine T.

"The attention to detail I receive when I come here is amazing. It's not a one size fits all approach. They look at each of my issues and take their time going thru each one, I don't feel like I'm being rushed in our out, I feel like I matter, and that's a great feeling."

–Austin H.

"What an amazing experience; and to think: people still take synthetic medicine for chiropractic pain? No need. This is the future. This is next. I look forward to coming back!"

–Evan T.

"Cryotherapy has decreased my down time and soreness between workouts. The staff and the doctor are extremely helpful and accommodating. I've never had to wait and every visit is engaging and I learn something new. Strongly recommend."

–Raouf I.

"Cryotherapy has decreased my down time and soreness between workouts. The staff and the doctor are extremely helpful and accommodating. I've never had to wait and every visit is engaging and I learn something new. Strongly recommend."

–Shawna O.

"Dr. Abraham and Angelica make this a great place to come for treatment. 5 stars!"

–Verry D.

"Amazing experience, came in and Dr. Robert knew exactly what to do! My pain was relieved in minutes! Highly recommend this facility! Going to CryoNext integrative healthcare was the best decision I've ever made to relieve my muscle pain!"

–George Y.

"Dr. Abraham and CryoNext have been pretty great. Their staff was very helpful and discerning. I'd recommend to anyone looking for a chiropractor. They also have all the latest and coolest tech in sports recovery. Really glad to have found them."

–Michael R.

"This place is awesome!!! I have been coming here at least once a week for the last 3 months to use the normatec compression sleeves. I have noticed that because the normatec helps relieve my sore muscles & joint, I'm able to recover faster & hit the gym harder. All the staff have been wonderful. easy to talk to, knowledgeable, and helpful."

– Eric N.

"I have had neuropathy for 27 years and I thought there was no way to recover from that until I came to see Dr. Abraham. The program was beyond my expectations. I have restored feeling in my hands and feet. I have no more pain, no hot and cold sensations, no pins and needles. I can sleep through the night. Dr. Abraham has helped me get my life back. Thank you."

–Gordon E.

"I have gone from 67% sensory loss in my feet to 2% in less than 90 days. I also had neuropathy in my hands to the point that I could not fill out my patient application legibly. I can now write with ease, no more numbness or pain in my hands or feet. This program has changed my life. I would recommend it to anyone who has neuropathy."

–Juan F.

"I have lost 16 lbs since starting the neuropathy program with Dr. Abraham. My blood glucose levels have significantly decreased. I was able to reduce my diabetes medication. I have also witnessed an improvement in my blood pressure readings and I am only half way through the program. Can't wait to see what I will look like at the end of the program."

––Angela F.

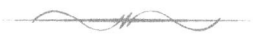

Bibliography

1. Go AS, Mozaffarian D, Roger VL, Benjamin EJ, Berry JD, Borden WB, Bravata DM, Dai S, Ford ES, Fox CS, Franco S, Fullerton HJ, Gillespie C, Hailpern SM, Heit JA, Howard VJ, Huffman MD, Kissela BM, Kittner SJ, Lackland DT, Lichtman JH, Lisabeth LD, Magid D, Marcus GM, Marelli A, Matchar DB, McGuire DK, Mohler ER, Moy CS, Mussolino ME, Nichol G, Paynter NP, Schreiner PJ, Sorlie PD, Stein J, Turan TN, Virani SS, Wong ND, Woo D, Turner MB; on behalf of the American Heart Association Statistics Committee and Stroke Statistics Subcommittee. Heart disease and stroke statistics—2013 update: a report from the American Heart Association.Circulation.2013;127:e6-e245.
2. Masters, Ryan, PhD. News. Columbia University Mailman School of Public Health. "Obesity Kills More Americans Than Previously Thought". N.p., 15 Aug. 2013.
3. Kochanek KD, Xu JQ, Murphy SL, Miniño AM, Kung HC. Deaths: final data for 2009. Adobe PDF file [PDF-2M] National vital statistics reports. 2011; 60(3).
4. Heidenreich PA, Trogdon JG, Khavjou OA, et al. Forecasting the future of cardiovascular disease in the United States: a policy statement from the American

Heart Association. Circulation. 2011;123:933-44. Epub 2011 Jan 24.

5. Go AS, Mozaffarian D, Roger VL, Benjamin EJ, Berry JD, Borden WB, Bravata DM, Dai S, Ford ES, Fox CS, Franco S, Fullerton HJ, Gillespie C, Hailpern SM, Heit JA, Howard VJ, Huffman MD, Kissela BM, Kittner SJ, Lackland DT, Lichtman JH, Lisabeth LD, Magid D, Marcus GM, Marelli A, Matchar DB, McGuire DK, Mohler ER, Moy CS, Mussolino ME, Nichol G, Paynter NP, Schreiner PJ, Sorlie PD, Stein J, Turan TN, Virani SS, Wong ND, Woo D, Turner MB; on behalf of the American Heart Association Statistics Committee and Stroke Statistics Subcommittee. Heart disease and stroke statistics—2013 update: a report from the American Heart Association.Circulation.2013;127:e6-e245.

6. Go AS, Mozaffarian D, Roger VL, Benjamin EJ, Berry JD, Borden WB, Bravata DM, Dai S, Ford ES, Fox CS, Franco S, Fullerton HJ, Gillespie C, Hailpern SM, Heit JA, Howard VJ, Huffman MD, Kissela BM, Kittner SJ, Lackland DT, Lichtman JH, Lisabeth LD, Magid D, Marcus GM, Marelli A, Matchar DB, McGuire DK, Mohler ER, Moy CS, Mussolino ME, Nichol G, Paynter NP, Schreiner PJ, Sorlie PD, Stein J, Turan TN, Virani SS, Wong ND, Woo D, Turner MB; on behalf of the American Heart Association Statistics Committee and Stroke Statistics Subcommittee. Heart disease and stroke statistics—2013 update: a report from the American Heart Association.Circulation.2013;127:e6-e245.

7. American Cancer Society. Cancer Facts & Figures 2013. Atlanta: American Cancer Society; 2013.

8. "Diabetes Statistics." Diabetes Basics. American Diabetes Association, 2013.

9. "Osteoporosis." NIHSeniorHealth.

10. Chris L. Peterson, Rachel Burton.The U.S. Health Care Spending. 2008.

11. Kane, Jason. "Health Costs: How the U.S. Compares With Other Countries." PBS. PBS, 22 Oct. 2012. Web.

12. "News Release." USDA Celebrates National Farmers Market Week, August 4-10. United States Department of Agriculture, 5 Aug. 2013. Web. 02 Aug. 2015. http://www.usda.gov/wps/portal/usda/usdahome?contentid=2013%2F08%2F0155.xml.

13. "Office of Public and Intergovernmental Affairs." News Releases - VA Office of Public and Intergovernmental Affairs, 25 Feb. 2014. Web. 02 Aug. 2015. http://www.va.gov/opa/pressrel/pressrelease.cfm?id=2529.

14. Eisenberg, DM, Kessler, RC, et al. New England Journal Medicine, "Unconventional Medicine in the United States -- Prevalence, Costs, and Patterns of Use." 1993.

15. Swift, Art. "Half of Americans Take Vitamins Regularly." Gallup.com. N.p., 19 Dec. 2013. Web. 02 Aug. 2015. http://www.gallup.com/poll/166541/half-americans-vitamins-regularly.aspx.

16. Who Killed Health Care?: America's $2 Trillion Medical Problem - and the Consumer-Driven Cure, Regina Herzlinger, 2007.

17. Mayo Clinic Staff. "Peripheral Neuropathy." Causes. Mayo Clinic, 04 Dec. 2014. Web. 22 July 2015. http://www.mayoclinic.org/diseases-conditions/peripheral-neuropathy/basics/causes/CON-20019948.

18. "The ReBuilder® Stops Pain While Treating Your Nerves - at Home." Safe, Effective Neuropathy Treatment. Web. 25 July 2015. http://www.rebuildermedical.com/.

19. Avci, P., Gupta, A., Sadasivam, M., Vecchio, D., Pam, Z., Pam, N., & Hamblin, M. R. (2013). Low-level laser (light) therapy (LLLT) in skin: stimulating, healing, restoring.

Seminars in Cutaneous Medicine and Surgery, 32(1), 41–52.

20. "Frequently Asked Questions." Frequently Asked Questions. Web. 25 July 2015. http://www. rebuildermedical.com/frequently-asked-questions.php#chemo.

21. Loghmani MT, Warden SJ. "Instrument-assisted cross-fiber massage accelerates knee ligament healing." Journal of Orthopaedic Sports Physical Therapy. 2009.

22. LeBauer A, Brtalik R, Stowe K. "The effect of myofascial release (MFR) on an adult with idiopathic scoliosis." Journal of Bodywork and Movement Therapies. 2008.

23. J BodywMovTher. 2013 Oct;17(4):518-22. doi: 10.1016/j. jbmt.2013.03.001. Epub 2013 Apr 30. http://www.ncbi. nlm.nih.gov/pubmed/24139013.

24. "Why Use VibePlate for Vibration Therapy, Vibration Traning, & Vibration Exercise." Why Use VibePlate for Vibration Therapy, Vibration Traning, & Vibration Exercise. N.p., n.d. Web. 26 July 2015. http://www. vibeplate.net/why-vibeplate.

25. MedlinePlus (June 7, 2012). U.S. National Library of Medicine. Medline Plus Trusted Health Information for You. Beta-carotene. Retrieved from www.nlm.nih.gov/ medlineplus/druginfo/natural/999.html.

26. LL Magnetic Clay Inc.(1996-2010). Ancient Minerals: Need More Magnesium? 10 Signs to Watch For. Retrieved from: www.ancient-minerals.com/ magnesium-deficiency/need-more/.

27. WebMD.(2005–2012). Weight Loss & Diet Plans. Top 10 Iron-Rich Foods. Retrieved from: www.webmd.com/ diet/features/top-10-iron-rich-foods.

28. More, J. (Sept. 2008). The British Dietetic Association. Vitamin D- The Unique Vitamin. Retrieved from: www. bda.uk.com/foodfacts/VitaminD.pdf.

29. Ferreira, Leonor Mateus. "Chiropractic Care May Help Control Peripheral Neuropathy in Diabetics." Diabetes News Journal. N.p., 16 Mar. 2015. Web. 27 July 2015. http://diabetesnewsjournal.com/2015/03/17/chiropractic-care-may-help-control-peripheral-neuropathy-in-diabetics/.

30. Medical Research Council. Regenerative medicine & stem cells. https://www.mrc.ac.uk/research/initiatives/regenerative-medicine-stem-cells.

31. Androutsellis-Theotokis A, Rueger MA, Park DM, et al. (August 2009). "Targeting neural precursors in the adult brain rescues injured dopamine neurons". Proc. Natl. Acad. Sci. U.S.A. 106 (32): 13570–75. https://www.ncbi.nlm.nih.gov/pubmed/19628689.

32. Team co-headed by researchers at Chosun University, Seoul National University and the Seoul Cord Blood BankArchived 1 May 2007 at the Wayback Machine. (SCB) Umbilical cord cells 'allow paralysed woman to walk' By Roger Highfield, Science Editor.

33. Ptaszek LM, Mansour M, Ruskin JN, Chien KR (2012). "Towards regenerative therapy for cardiac disease". The Lancet. 379 (9819): 933–42. doi:10.1016/s0140-6736(12)60075-0.

34. Fetal tissue restores lost sight. MedicalNewsToday. 28 October 2004. https://www.medicalnewstoday.com/releases/15535.php.

35. Goldstein, Ron (2007). Embryonic stem cell research is necessary to find a diabetes cure. Greenhaven Press. p. 44.

36. Rosemann A (Dec 2014). "Why regenerative stem cell medicine progresses slower than expected". J Cell Biochem. 115 (12): 2073–76. https://www.ncbi.nlm.nih.gov/pubmed/25079695.

37. Wikipedia. Platelet-rich plasma. https://en.wikipedia.org/wiki/Platelet-rich_plasma.

38. Rabago, D; Nourani, B (2017). "Prolotherapy for Osteoarthritis and Tendinopathy: a Descriptive Review". Current Rheumatology Reports. 19 (6): 34. doi:10.1007/s11926-017-0659-3.

39. Bauer, Brent A. (2012). "Prolotherapy: Solution to low back pain?". Mayo Clinic. Retrieved 16 December 2012.

40. Distel, Laura M.; Best, Thomas M. (2011). "Prolotherapy: A Clinical Review of Its Role in Treating Chronic Musculoskeletal Pain". PM&R. 3 (6): S78–81. https://www.ncbi.nlm.nih.gov/pubmed/21703585.

41. Rabago, D; Slattengren, A; Zgierska, A (2010). "Prolotherapy in Primary Care Practice". Primary Care: Clinics in Office Practice. 37 (1): 65–80. https://www.ncbi.nlm.nih.gov/pubmed/20188998.

42. Banks, AR (1991). "A Rationale for Prolotherapy" (PDF). Journal of Orthopaedic Medicine. 13 (3).

43. Judson, Christopher H.; Wolf, Jennifer Moriatis (2013). "Lateral Epicondylitis". Orthopedic Clinics of North America. 44 (4): 615–23. https://www.ncbi.nlm.nih.gov/pubmed/24095076.

44. Covey, CJ; Sineath, MH Jr; Penta, JF; Leggit, JC (2015). "Prolotherapy: Can it help your patient?". Journal of Family Practice. 64 (12): 763–768. https://www.ncbi.nlm.nih.gov/pubmed/26844994.

45. Distel, Laura M.; Best, Thomas M. (2011). "Prolotherapy: A Clinical Review of Its Role in Treating Chronic

Musculoskeletal Pain". PM&R. 3 (6): S78–81. https://www.ncbi.nlm.nih.gov/pubmed/21703585.

46. Lombardi, G., Ziemann, E., & Banfi, G. (2017). Whole-Body Cryotherapy in Athletes: From Therapy to Stimulation. An Updated Review of the Literature. Frontiers in Physiology, 8, 258. http://doi.org/10.3389/fphys.2017.00258.

47. Banfi G, Lombardi G, Colombini A, and Melegati G. Whole-Body Cryotherapy in Athletes. Sports Med 2010; doi: 10.2165/11531940-000000000-00000 0112-1642/10/0000-0000/$49.95/0.

48. Pournot H, Bieuzen F, Louis J, Fillard J-R, Barbiche E, et al. (2011) Time-Course of Changes in Inflammatory Response after Whole-Body Cryotherapy Multi Exposures following Severe Exercise. PLoS ONE 6(7): e22748. doi:10.1371/journal.pone.0022748.

49. Hausswirth C, Louis J, Bieuzen F, Pournot H, Fournier J, et al. (2011) Effects of Whole-Body Cryotherapy vs. Far-Infrared vs. Passive Modalities on Recovery from Exercise-Induced Muscle Damage in Highly-Trained Runners PLoS ONE 6(12): e27749. doi:10.1371/journal.pone.0027749.

50. Ziemann E, Antoni R, Kujach S, Grzywacz T, et al. (2012) Five-Day Whole-Body Cryostimulation, Blood Inflammatory Markers, and Performance in High-Ranking Professional Tennis Players. Journal of Athletic Training 2012;47(6):664–672 doi: 10.4085/1062-6050-47.6.13.

51. Metzger D, Zwingmann C, Protz W, Jäckel WH. (2000) Whole-body cryotherapy in rehabilitation of patients with rheumatoid diseases--pilot study. Rehabilitation (Stuttg). 2000 Apr;39(2):93-100.

52. Rymaszewska J, Ramsey D. Whole body cryotherapy as a novel adjuvant therapy for depression and anxiety. Archives of Psychiatry and Psychotherapy, 2008; 2 : 49–57.

53. Apfel et al., Restoration of disk height through non-surgical spinal decompression is associated with decreased discogenic low back pain: a retrospective cohort study. BMC Musculoskeletal Disorders 2010, 11:155.

54. Beattie et al. Short and long term outcomes following treatment with the VAX-D for patients with chronic, activity-limiting low back pain. Journal of Orthopedic and Sports Physical Therapy 2005 (Volume 35, Number 1).

55. Ramos, G. Efficacy of vertebral axial decompression on chronic low back pain: study of dosage regimen. Journal of Neurologic Research 2004 (Volume 26, Number 3).

56. Mayo Clinic. Hyperbaric Oxygen Therapy. https://www.mayoclinic.org/tests-procedures/hyperbaric-oxygen-therapy/about/pac-20394380.

57. Boussi-Gross R, Golan H, Fishlev G, Bechor Y, Volkov O, Bergan J, et al. (2013) Hyperbaric Oxygen Therapy Can Improve Post Concussion Syndrome Years after Mild Traumatic Brain Injury - Randomized Prospective Trial. PLoS ONE 8(11): e79995. doi:10.1371/journal.pone.0079995.

58. Efrati, S., Fishlev, G., Bechor, Y., Volkov, O., Bergan, J., Kliakhandler, K., Kamiager, I., Gal, N., Friedman, M., Ben-Jacob, E., & Golan, H. (2013). Hyperbaric Oxygen Induces Late Neuroplasticity in Post Stroke Patients – Randomized, Prospective Trial. PLoS ONE, 8(1): e53716 doi: 10.1371/journal.pone.0053716.

59. Mayo Clinic. Knee Pain. https://www.mayoclinic.org/
diseases-conditions/knee-pain/symptoms-causes/
syc-20350849.

60. Mayo Clinic. Plantar-Fasciitis. https://www.mayoclinic.
org/diseases-conditions/plantar-fasciitis/diagnosis
-treatment/drc-20354851.

61. George Dvorsky. The Switch to Outdoor LED Lighting
Has Completely Backfired. https://gizmodo.com/
the-switch-to-outdoor-led-lighting-has-completely-
backf-1820652615.

62. Ezra Klein. The American Prospect. Ten Reasons Why
American Health Care Is so Bad. http://prospect.org/
article/ten-reasons-why-american-health-care-so-bad.

63. Dr. Mercola. March 15, 2014. Top Ten Ways the American
Health Care System Fails.http://articles.mercola.com/
sites/articles/archive/2014/03/15/bad-american-
health-care-system.aspx#_edn16.

64. Roberts R.O. et al. (2015, May 5.) Risk and protective
factors for cognitive impairment in persons aged 85
years and older. Neurology, 84, 18, 1854-61.

65. The University of Arizona Center of Integrative
Medicine. What is Integrative Medicine? https://
integrativemedicine.arizona.edu/about/definition.html